First USA Edition

ISBN: 978-0-9894801-1-6

Front and Back Cover Illustration: Katie Rabitor

KAROLINA LABRECQUE

For my husband, best friend and biggest supporter Michael and daughter Magda, both stars in my universe.

Table of Contents

FOREWORD

"I want to get a horse!" my sister would often plead with my parents. It seemed like the most important thing she could do. Many Sunday drives were punctuated by looking at horses grazing by the side of the road. In additional to being common for girls to want a horse perhaps my sister also sensed getting in the saddle would be good for her younger brother with autism.

My first time on a horse was scary. After climbing into what seemed to be an impossible high saddle the leader told me to hold on to the reins and wait. Perhaps the same problems in visual perception causing me to run away from a baseball being gently tossed to me by my father in a game of catch accentuated the height and seeming peril of sitting on a (proverbial) high horse! I must have held the reins too short and tight because the horse kept shifting his weight, moving his head, and smuttering. We hadn't even started to head out to the paddocks and I had to get off the horse.

However, things could have been better. This gift of a resource to the autism community from Dr. LaBrecque will introduce you to the world of intervention for people with autism and other disabilities through myriad techniques available through Equine Assisted Activities and Therapies (EAAT). For example, had there been a certified Therapeutic Horseback Riding (THR) instructor available I would have had a much easier time with the animal. Many years later, I visited a therapeutic riding farm in Kentucky having a THR made saddling up and riding the horse a very enjoyable experience.

With the expertise of a scientist based on her own research conducted on the efficacy of EAAT, Karolina explains in easy to understand terms what autism is – and in particular the neurobiological differences current research informs us about in the condition. This foundation of understanding about autism is used to launch artistically described well known techniques and approaches for working with individuals on the autism spectrum and addressing challenging behaviors that may occur within the context of hippotherapy sessions.

Some of these techniques and methods described within the context of EAAT include sensory integration therapy Applied Behavior Analysis (ABA), Developmental Individual Difference Relationship-Based Intervention (DIR), the Miller Method (MM), Relational Development Intervention (RDI), Treatment and Education of Autistic and Communication Handicapped Children (TEACCH), Social Communication Emotional Regulations Transactional Support Model (SCERTS), and the Son Rise program (SR).

The groundbreaking aspect of Dr. LeBrecques' work is in her skillful alignment of specific examples where aspects of EAAT can be implemented within the context of each of these approaches. Here the focus is on matching intervention to individual needs. *Healing Horses* is a must read for anyone desiring to know more about the therapeutic role horses can play for enabling those on the autism spectrum to lead fulfilling and productive lives to their greatest potential.

Stephen Shore, Ed.D.

Clinical Assistant Professor of Special Education at Adelphi University

Internationally known author, consultant, and presenter on issues related to the autism spectrum

Introduction

In 2010, the center for Disease Control estimated that 1 in 68 children had been identified as having some form of Autism Spectrum Disorder. Even though the precise cause of autism has yet to be identified, one can find many forms of therapy offered to both children and adults who live with this condition. While some of these therapies are widely known, extensively researched, and described in great detail; others, such as the use of horses in the therapeutic process have little more than anecdotal proof and are not completely understood.

If you have picked up this book, you are likely a horse enthusiast, therapist, or know someone who has been diagnosed with autism and are curious as to the role the horse can play in therapy. This book has been written as an attempt to demystify the influence of a horse on a person (especially a child) living with ASD. It is addressed to parents, caregivers, EAAT therapist, and future EAAT professionals. It is an attempt to show the both the science and practical application of using the horse as a therapeutic tool for an autistic child. . For those readers familiar with the EAAT knowledge, it is an attempt at a practical guide of the most popular approaches to autism. The information in this book includes the more than 15 years of practical experience I have as a hippotherapist and therapeutic horseback riding instructor, as well as thoroughly researched and supported knowledge from additional sources.

In Part One –The Magic of The Horse- you will find basic information about the EAAT industry and how the horse influences the human being. Part Two provides an overview of ASD. Part Three will walk you through the most common therapeutic approaches to autism. Finally, Part Four will show how the horse can specifically help a child with autism. Each section of this book can be used independent of one another, or use as whole to provide a comprehensive overview.

I hope you enjoy.

Karolina LaBrecque, PhD

PART ONE

THE MAGIC OF THE HORSE

CHAPTER ONE

History of the Horse in Medicine

From the beginning of humanity the life of people interweaved with existence of horses. From the time of Upper Paleolithic[1] we can find paintings of horses[2] on the walls of caves and other hiding places where people were living. They were first considered by humans as game animals. Primitive men hunted horses, ate their meat, and used their skin (as clothing) and bones (as tools) (Wyżnikiewicz Nawracała, 2002).

Five thousand years ago, somewhere in Asia humans started to domesticate horses. They were first used by the nomads for transportation (of both people and goods) and as source of meat and milk (Grabowski, 1982). With progression of military tactics after agricultural communities emerged, horses became even more appreciated. The domesticated horses, in addition to their use in the army, replaced the earlier used donkey and ox in agriculture and transportation. (Grabowski, 1982)

In some culture horses had a very special position and different myths were created around them. After all, the horse served humans in many different and essential ways. In addition of using the horse for combat, transportation, and in agriculture people also noticed therapeutic benefits of this animal very early on. Horseback rid-

---

[1] The Upper Paleolithic (or Upper Palaeolithic, and also in some contexts *Late Stone Age*) is the third and last subdivision of the Paleolithic or Old Stone Age as it is understood in Europe, Africa and Asia. Very broadly it dates to between 40,000 and 10,000 years ago, roughly coinciding with the appearance of behavioral modernity and before the advent of agriculture. The terms "Late Stone Age" and "Upper Paleolithic" refer to the same periods. For historical reasons, "Stone Age" usually refers to the period in Africa, whereas "Upper Paleolithic" is generally used when referring to the period in Europe. (http://en.wikipedia.org/wiki/Upper_Paleolithic)

[2] So far the oldest discovered paintings where made about 20000 years ago.

ing started to be used as a means of therapy in the V Century B.C. (Wyżnikiewicz Nawracała, 2002). It was employed to rehabilitate wounded soldiers (Biery, 1985). Later, horseback riding was prescribed by philosophers, scientist and medics as exercise for both the body and the mind (ex. Socrates 469-399 B.C, Awicenna 980-1037).

The development of therapeutic horseback riding in the XX Century was strongly influenced by spectacular success of Danish rider Liz Hartel. Even though she had polio, she participated in dressage competitions and in 1952 she won the silver medal in dressage at the Olympic Games. In 1954, largely based on the success of Hartel, Norah Jacques introduced hippotherapy as part of her work with children with movement disorders. From then on therapy with the use of a horse became more and more popular and slowly started to spread from Canada and North America to the rest of the world.

At the beginning hippotherapy was used for children with different movement disabilities of various origins. Later it was gradually introduced as supplement to rehabilitation of other types of disabilities in children and in adults. Currently it is utilized among others in cases of cerebral palsy, in rehabilitation of people with amputations, the blind, people with psychomotor problems, spasticity, congestive heart failure, microcephaly, multiple sclerosis, and problems with postures. Equine Assisted Activities and Therapies (EAAT) are also used for patients with mental problems (depression, schizophrenia, substance abuse etc) and developmental problems. Therapists and parents notice that horse has a positive influence on people with autism, Down Syndrome, mental retardation, behavioral problems, alcoholism, depression, injuries to CNS, and personality disorders.

From the above we can see that the field of EAAT moved from simple therapeutic riding or different versions of exercise on the horse to a very broad field with many different modalities and specialties. Each country uses a slightly different system of classification and division of EAAT. The language and classifications very often depend on the local laws governing medical and paramedical practice and the license for recreational and sport trainers. Below is the description of the system proposed by the PATH International which is a non- profit organization governing the development of EAAT in USA.

CHAPTER TWO

What is EAAT

Equine Assisted Activities and Therapies (EAAT) are all activities that utilize a horse for the purpose of contributing positively to the cognitive, physical, emotional and social well being of people with disabilities. (PATH International, 2011). There are many forms of EAAT. Some of them involve riding, others just spending time with the horses or being around them (un-mounted activities). EAAT include therapies, recreation, and high level sport competitions. Below is a short description of each of the forms of EAAT.

Hippotherapy
Hippotherapy is any form of therapy that utilizes the horse as a life therapeutic tool. The goals and activities for hippotherapy are the same as for any other therapy. The client exercises on the horse and does not steer or direct the horse. The sessions are always provided by a licensed therapist. In the USA, hippotherapy treatment is provided by an occupational or physical therapist or speech and language pathologist who must additionally be certified by the AHA[3]. If the therapist is not PATH INTERNATIONAL certified, a PATH INTERNATIONAL certified instructor responsible for the horse behavior should be also present during the session.

Equine Facilitated Psychotherapy
This form of therapy can be provided by a licensed mental health specialist. Therapy session can be done on a horse or off the horse. Depending on the form of the class it can be provided either by a therapist who is certified as a THR instructor (for mounted sessions) or in the case of un-mounted session (sessions that do not involve riding the horse) by a therapist with an Equine Specialist in Mental Health and Learning Certification.

---

3 AHA (American Hippotherapy Association)

Equine facilitated learning

Equine facilitated learning utilizes experiential learning, also known as "learning by doing", to promote the development and growth of participants. During the sessions participants interact with the environment (people, animals, etc.) and get involved in different scenarios. Each participant has different goals (for example improving social skills, behavior management, self-care skills, etc.). During sessions, students learn about themselves, about horses, their environment, and build skills that can be transferred to everyday life. The sessions are supervised by professionals within the educational field and can take place on or off the horse. Participants learn through observing and interacting with the horses but also during other activities (coloring books, journaling, goal setting, learning about horse, and horseback riding theory, etc.).

Therapeutic horseback riding (THR)

THR is a form of EAAT that involves active horseback riding. During THR participants learn how to ride a horse in a safe and supervised manner. Depending on their situation they can ride independently or with full supervision. Very often the horse is directly overseen by a leader on the ground and the person is accompanied by side-walker or two, whose role is to ensure safety and give the rider support that may be needed. The lessons can be individual or in groups, depending on the need of the participant(s). A qualified instructor should always be present during the lesson[4]. The lesson can take place in a variety of different environments. The rider can stay in an enclosed arena, indoor arena (especially during bad weather) or go on trail rides. The goal of THR is to allow the participant to gain as much independent riding skill as possible and at the same time to incorporate therapeutic goals that can be helpful in other aspects of life. Well-structured THR programs are supervised by a group of clinicians consisting of an occupational therapist, physical therapist, speech

---

[4] In the USA there is no requirement by law that a therapeutic horseback riding instructor have any special certification. However an instructor that is serious about teaching THR in a safe and professional manner will be PATH INTERNATIONAL certified and the center will have PATH INTERNATIONAL accreditation or membership.

therapist, and sometimes also a psychologist. In the case of children the goals from IEP are very often incorporated into the riding goals. The natural progression for THR is participation in equine sports.

SPORT

Special Olympics

Special Olympics[5] is the world's largest sport organization for children and adults with intellectual disabilities, providing year-round training and competitions to more than 3.1 million athletes in 175 countries. In equestrian sports qualifying competitions and state shows/championships are held. Participants can train and show on club horses or have they own. The riders compete at different levels which they are assigned depending on their ability to safely negotiate any movements required in the given class and they compete according to ability and age. There are 3 general Levels of competition:

Level A - Walk/Trot/Jog Center/Lope- independent only. The rider is expected to compete with no modification to general rules.

Level B- Walk and Trot/Jog

Level C- Walk only

The above levels are broken down to even more specific groups. The competitions are held in Dressage, Prix Caprilli, English Equitation, Western Equitation, Western Riding, Working Trails, Showmanship, Team Relays, Pole Bending, Barrel Racing, Figure 8 Stake Race, and Drill Team of 2 or 4 horses.

Paralympics

The Paralympics are the highest level of participation in adapted activity sports that an athlete with any kind of challenges can enter without having to compete in the main stream sports. They are the elite sport events for athletes with a disability. They emphasize, however, the participants' athletic achievements rather than their disability.

---

[5] If you are interest more about learning about the whole Special Olympic movement, traditions and history please visit http://www.specialolympics.org/.

In the case of equestrian sports right now only dressage and carriage driving competitions are held. Competitors are classified as a team horse/rider (or driver).

If you have a permanent, measurable disability you may compete in ParaEquestrian Classes. PE Classes are held at either FEI/USEF PE shows (for riders with a disability) or at open USEF/USDF shows. Each rider has his physical abilities evaluated and is assigned a classification. The assessed impairment and the resulting functional profile are compared with other profiles that should have similar ability when mounted. Classification is a structure for competition. Paralympics athletes have an impairment in body structures and functions that leads to a competitive disadvantage in sport. Consequently, criteria are put in place to ensure that winning is determined by skill, fitness, power, endurance, tactical ability and mental focus, the same factors that account for success in sport for athletes who are able-bodied.

There are four groups of classification in dressage:

Gr1. Mainly for wheelchair users with poor trunk balance and or impairment in all four limbs, or no trunk balance and good upper limb function, or moderate trunk balance with severe impairment of all four limbs. This group competes at a level equivalent to USDF Intro Level.

Gr 2. Mainly wheelchair users, or those with severe locomotor impairment involving the trunk and with good to mild upper limb function, those with severe arm impairment and slight leg impairment or severe unilateral impairments. This group is equivalent to USEF Training Level.

Gr. 3. Participants usually able to walk without support. Moderate unilateral impairment, or moderate impairment in four limbs, severe arm impairment. Many need a wheelchair for longer distances or due to lack of stamina. Total loss of sight in both eyes, or intellectually impaired. This group competes at equivalent to USEF First Level.

Gr. 4. Impairment in one or two limbs or some visual impairment. Participant competes at the level equivalent to USEF Third Level.

The Carriage Driving is divided into two groups:

Gr. 1. For wheelchair users with poor trunk balance and impairment in upper limbs, or those who are able to walk, but with impairment of function in all four limbs, or those with severe arm impairment only.

Gr. 2. Those with less impairment than Grade I yet are functionally disadvantaged against able bodied drivers.

We will look at the therapeutic driving in the next section.

Therapeutic Driving

"Therapeutic Carriage Driving can offer students with physical, mental, sensory, or emotional disabilities the rewards of interaction and control of a horse or pony while driving from a carriage seat or in their own wheelchair in a carriage modified to accommodate their wheelchair."[6] Driving provides a good alternative for those who are unable to participate in riding lessons for many different reasons. The most common reasons may include inability to sit, weight, luck of balance, allergies, fear of heights etc. Therapeutic driving is based on team work and teaches safety, basic horsemanship skills, harnessing and driving skills. Participants improve their social/emotional, cognitive and physical abilities.

Interactive Vaulting

Equestrian vaulting is most often described as gymnastics and dance on horseback and, like these disciplines, it can be practiced as a non-competitive art or as a competitive sport.[7] Interactive Vaulting engag-

---

[6] http://www.horseshelpingpeoplema.com/eaa.html#efl
[7] http://en.wikipedia.org/wiki/Equestrian_vaulting

es participants in gymnastic while participating in horsemanship activities and learning to work as a team. It provides exercise and movement, educational opportunities, and social interaction. The activities may include caring for and handling the horses, exercise on a barrel, exercise on a standing still or moving horse. When in motion the horse is trained to move in a circle on a lunge line (a long leash for a horse) controlled by an instructor. Students start with simple positions like sitting facing forward, sideway or backwards and slowly progress to more complicated movements such as kneeling or standing on the horse. Sessions are structured as group lessons with emphasis on the individual needs of each participant. The sessions are directed by an instructor who should be certified in Interactive Vaulting.

CHAPTER THREE

So how does EAAT works?

So how exactly does the horse influence the human? The biggest magic of the horse-human relationship is that the horse can influence participants in many dimensions at the same time. Thirty minutes of EAAT can have a positive effect on physical, emotional and social development. In one lesson the therapist can address sensory needs, work on physical strength and social interaction, hand eye coordination, and add work with accordance with IEP. In this chapter I will show you the most common ways in which EAAT works.

General gates and their influence

Most mounted lessons (therapeutic horseback riding sessions and hippotherapy session) take place at 'walk'. The walk is a symmetrical four bit gait that averages 4 miles per hour. When walking, a horse's legs follow this sequence: left hind leg, left front leg, right hind leg, right front leg, in a regular 1-2-3-4 beat. At the walk, the horse will always have one foot raised and the other three feet on the ground, save for a brief moment when weight is being transferred from one foot to another. A horse moves its head and neck in a slight up and down motion that helps maintain its balance. [8]

If the client is sitting on the horse correctly and facing forward at the walk he or she will experience movement in different planes. The back legs of the horse cause acceleration of the rider in the sagittal plane and their alternating reaching underneath the horse's trunk causes the rider to move up and down. The movement of the horse's legs on either the left or right side causes the rider to move in the frontal plane and the movement of horse's pelvis from side to side and forward rotates the pelvis of the rider[9]. All of the movements combined give the almost perfect simulation of the human walk.

---

[8] Harris, S., 1993
[9] Łojek, 2006

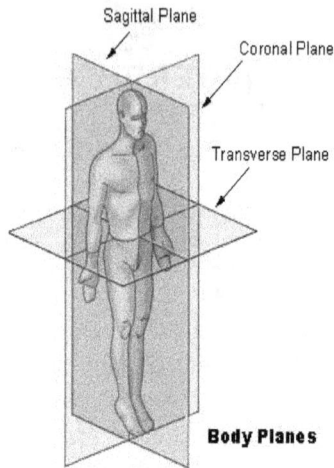

Sagittal Plane
Coronal Plane
Transverse Plane
Body Planes

The rider and the horse form a system. For that system to remain stable the center of gravity of the rider has to be placed above the center of the gravity of the horse[10]. The center of gravity of the horse during movement is constantly changing. When the horse is standing on all four legs it has a more or less rectangular base. Raising a front or a back leg changes the shape of the base into a triangle[11]. The center of gravity of the horse changes in the matter shown in Pic 2.

If we assume that the horse moves in an even, symmetrical four bit gait and that the client is a child who is passively sitting on the horse, not trying to direct its movement, we can assume that the difference of the body mass between a child and a horse will cause the horse to influence the center of gravity of the child and not the other way around.[12] It means that with every step of the horse the child has to rebalance itself. Just a passive seating on a moving horse engages the vestibular system, core muscle and body awareness.

The situation gets even more complicated in the case of an adult or when we start doing different exercises on the horse. By shifting the center of gravity the rider influences the horse which in turn adjusts its body forcing the rider to again shift his or her center of gravity.

---

[10] Clayton, 2004
[11] Clayton, 2004
[12,6] Przewloka K., 2007.

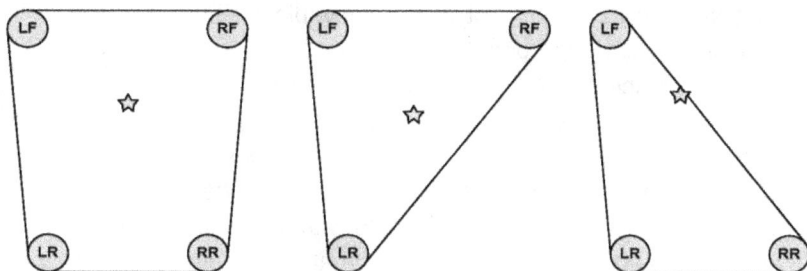

Pic 2. Change of the center of gravity in relation to the base. LR- left rear, LF left front, RR right rear, -, RF –right front.

Just like humans, horses come in different sizes and with different conformation (build). It is very important that the size of the horse, and the way it moves, are matched with the size of the client. Each client should be matched with a horse that not only has a proper barrel width, but also has the right length of the straight and amplitude of movement. If the horse is too large for a child it will not only be very uncomfortable to seat on, but will also provoke extensive movement of the lower back and pelvis, possibly putting strain on the muscular-skeletal system.

Higher level therapeutic riding lessons will also utilize trot and canter. The trot is a two-beat gait that has a wide variation in possible speeds, but averages about 8 miles per hour (13 km/h). Depending on the horse and its speed, a trot can be difficult for a rider to sit, because the body of the horse actually drops a bit between beats and bounces

up again when the next set of legs strike the ground. The body be-
haves like a bouncing ball and if one tenses up, just as in a case of a
well inflated ball, the bounce will be stronger. Sitting the trot requires
just the right amount of contraction of stomach muscle and relaxation
of back muscle. If one relaxes too much it will result in a loss of balance and control over the horse. Tense up and you become a bouncing ball. To make the trot more enjoyable for both the rider and the
horse long time ago people came up with the idea of posting. Posting
involves rising out of the saddle seat for every other stride of the horses' forelegs. It is never used in hippotherapy, but can be used in advanced therapeutic horseback riding lessons. It requires a lot of
coordination on the part of the rider, because the lower leg from knee
down stays motionless and the hips with the torso move forward. The
hands should not move at all. All of that is executed in harmony to the
horse's movement.

The Trot can be executed with a leader and side-walkers, on a lounge
line or off the line. Before attempting to trot independently, the rider
should first be able to demonstrate ability to stop, turn and get the
horse moving at the walk and maintain balance during the trot while
on the lunge line.

The last gait that I would like to discus is canter. Riding the canter is
reserved only for the most advanced clients and can be done on a
lounge line or off line. Canter is a controlled, three-beat gait that usually is a bit faster than the average trot. The average speed of a canter
is between 16–27 km/h (10–17 mph). In the canter, one of the horse's
rear legs – the right rear leg, for example – propels the horse forward.
During this beat, the horse is supported only on that single leg while
the remaining three legs are moving forward. On the next beat the
horse catches itself on the left rear and right front legs while the other
hind leg is still momentarily on the ground. On the third beat, the horse
catches itself on the left front leg while the diagonal pair is momentarily still in contact with the ground[13].

---

[13] Harris, Susan E. *Horse Gaits, Balance and Movement* New York: Howell
Book House 1993 p. 42-44

To be able to pick up safe, slow canter and to maintain it, the rider has to use asymmetrical aids and be able to follow the horses movement all of the time. Some horses can also get a bit more excited in canter and want to go faster especially if the rider is off balance and is shifting the horse's center of gravity forward. All of the above make canter a much harder gait to control and to maintain.

Besides varying horses' gaits, a therapist can also influence the rider through leading the horse with different straight lengths and through corners. The longer the horse step, the bigger the amplitude of the rider's movement. A very good exercise for stabilizing the core muscles and building body awareness is stop and go. Every time the horse stops or starts moving the rider has to catch his or her balance and adjust body position.

Another challenging exercise is work on a circle. When the horse moves on the circle the rider experiences the centrifugal force. This force represents the effects of inertia that arise in connection with rotation and which are experienced as an outward force away from the center of rotation. When the horse is moving on a circle the rider has to counterbalance the centrifugal force by contracting his or her core muscle on the side of body that is closer to the inside of the circle. The smaller the circle the more work the horse and the rider have to do. The same rule applies when riding through a corner or through turns. The sharper the turn the more work has to be done by the muscles. For this reason it is very important to always work equally on both directions unless we are trying to correct postural imbalance by over-strengthening one side of the body while gently stretching the other side.

Now that we have a better understanding of the basic influence of the horse on the rider we can move on to more advanced benefits such as the improvement of sensory integration (described in chapter three), psychological effects, and education in general. Specific guidelines for the influence of EAAT in these areas on people on ASD are described in chapter four.

Psychosocial aspect of EAAT

Working with horses not only provides physical benefits but also has tremendous psychosocial influence. Just the pure fact that the therapy takes place at a barn, in a natural environment and outside of a typical therapeutic setting provides additional stimulation. The biggest attribute of the horse during therapy is that it provides a motivation and a non-judgmental environment. The EAAT activities are not perceived by a client as therapy, but as a time with a horse. Properly developed lessons and therapy sessions can have a very broad positive influence and can be incorporated into other activities outside of the barn setting.

Social development

The first thing that all clients should learn when starting EAAT participation is that there are rules that need to be followed. All the rules should be followed not only by clients, but also by parents, volunteers, staff, and care givers. The rules should be presented in a way that the client can understand. If one understands why something should be done or is not allowed to do, the chances of following a given rule increase. A simple 'no' or 'you must do it' may not be sufficient for the client to remember. The most common rules in the barn are: wearing a helmet while on a horse, no running or screaming in the barn, not approaching the horse from the behind, and no hand feeding the horse. All of the above are safety related and can be easily explained to the clients.

Learning to understand and follow the rules in the barn helps the client to follow the rules in everyday life and understand the consequences of breaking them.

Another aspect of social development is understanding body language and spatial relations. The horses can be very good teachers of that. Learning to read nonverbal cues from the horse and its way of communicating can help clients, especially clients with autism, pay more attention to the complex word of nonverbal communication in every day live.

Different forms of EAAT also allow for group activity. Group therapeutic riding sessions or volting are particularly appropriate for development of group cooperation, taking turns and giving support to each other.

Working in the group setting or individually with a therapist around horses provides a lot of opportunities for proper expression of one's needs. Therapists have to be prepared to deal with difficult behaviors and not allow them to escalate. Giving opportunities to express one's needs, allowing one to make choices, and teaching proper ways of expressing emotions can all take place on or around the horse.

Another form of group activities, which can be very beneficial for some clients, is the competitions. The set of rules, the preparation, and emotional charge of winning a ribbon take horseback riding goals to a much higher level. Taking part in Special Olympics, Para-Olympics or dressage competitions, showing the fruits of the hard work and preparation in front of judges, parents, and spectators has tremendous psychological value and influences self-esteem as well as locus of control. This leads us to the psychological benefits of EAAT.

Elements of psychotherapy during EAAT

Although one of the aims of EAAT is psychotherapy, the elements of it can be found during almost any activity with the horse. Starting EAAT sessions usually involves stepping into a totally new and unknown world of the horse and its surroundings. It is up to the instructor to build a positive relation with the client and to facilitate positive relation between the client and the horse. The horse, if treated right, will never criticize the client and will not judge. No matter what the abilities of the client, he or she will always feel welcome and accepted which in turn may influence their perception of self and self-acceptance.

Being able to control a big animal and having an opportunity to choose between different activities on the horse can also have tremendous influence on the locus of control[14] of our clients. Most children, but especially children with some kind of disability, have no control over what they do, and when they do it. Most are also not used to directing others. The same can be said about adults with mental disabilities or severe physical limitations. Being on the horse and directing its movements or controlling it from the ground can empower the clients and shift their locus of control to internal. It empowers and teaches them how do make decisions. It can also benefit their self-esteem. I strongly encourage all of the parents and care givers of children and clients that participate in EAAT to try at least once to get on the horse and do what our participants do. I can guarantee that, if you never rode before, your perspective on this activity and abilities that it requires will change tremendously[15]. One thing that you will notice is that at the very beginning being on a horse can be a scary experience. This brings us to another psychological aspect: the fear.

Dealing with Fear

In everyday life, most people seldom get to interact with animals as big and different as horses. Not knowing what to expect, not under-

---

[14] **Locus of control** is a theory in personality psychology referring to the extent to which individuals believe that they can control events that affect them. Understanding of the concept was developed by Julian B. Rotter in 1954, and has since become an important aspect of personality studies. One's "locus" (Latin for "place" or "location") can either be internal (meaning the person believes that they control their life) or external (meaning they believe that their environment, some higher power, or other people control their decisions and their life).Individuals with a high internal locus of control believe that events result primarily from their own behavior and actions. Those with a high external locus of control believe that powerful others, fate, or chance primarily determine events. Those with a high internal locus of control have better control of their behavior, tend, and are more likely to attempt to influence other people than those with a high external (or low internal respectively) locus of control. Those with a high internal locus of control are more likely to assume that their efforts will be successful. They are more active in seeking information and knowledge concerning their situation.
(http://en.wikipedia.org/wiki/Locus_of_control).

[15] If you do take up this challenge, please share your experience at thehealinghorses.com

standing body language and movement of the horse can be scary especially for people with limited cognitive abilities. All the sensory input and stimulation, the new surroundings and new situations provide an opportunity to face ones fears and learn how to deal with stress in new situations.

It is up to the therapist/instructor to set up the sessions in such a way that they are not overwhelming to the client. Gradual introduction of the horse and activities that allow a little bit of fear will lead to a trust-building relation with the horse and increase their self-esteem. On the other hand physically forcing a client to do something that they are afraid of can permanently discourage them from participating and should be avoided at all cost.

The fear can also be caused by separation from the care taker, or because the person does not have many opportunities to experience independence from others. In both of these cases EAAT can provide an excellent opportunity to overcome those road blocks, and learn new coping skill that can be incorporated into everyday life.

Connected to fear can be ability to express emotions. Very often EAAT clients have problems with expressing emotions in a socially accepted way. Sometimes they scream, hit the horse, the instructor, or side walkers. By explaining how the horse may react or showing the horse's reaction to those inappropriate means of expression, the EAAT team can help the client learn behaviors that are socially acceptable. Even nonverbal clients can be equipped with tools that will allow for acceptable expression. By giving someone tools to communicate we open the door to self-expression, lower frustration, and individual as well as social growth.

The moments in which a client can help another client take care of the horse play a very important role in the development of social growth. Group lesson and un-mounted activities, like grooming and feeding, are all excellent opportunities for empowering the person to be independent. The ability to help others in the life of a person that very often requires a lot of help can have tremendous positive effect and open new possibilities in everyday life.

Elements of special education:

EAAT in most cases is an additional form of therapy and should complement all other interventions and activities in the client's life. A well designed EAAT program incorporates collaboration between specialists and parents. Sessions can be structured so that clients can implement the themes learned in a different setting. For example trail rides can be utilized to talk about different seasons and colors. Counting cons/toys, etc. can show practical application of math. "Scavenger Hunt" games and "maps" can provide opportunities to learn new vocabulary and reinforce what was previously learned.

Elements of speech therapy:

One of the forms of EAAT hippotherapy allows speech therapist to use the horse as a therapeutic tool. Elements of speech therapy can be incorporated into many forms of EAAT if needed, however. Below are some examples of speech therapy exercises that can be done on the horse.

-*Breathing exercises* (like blowing a leaf or grass out of the horse's mane, taking in deep a breath in with a toy on the stomach and breathing out to see if the toy will rise up and down, etc.)

-*Recognition of sounds from the surroundings* (recognition of the sound of hoofs on different sources, sounds of different animals that can be found on the farm, etc.)

-*Reacting to sounds* (the therapist can utilize different games to teach the client to react to a sound that was previously introduced both to the child and to the horse)

-*Understanding verbal commands* (As in any other situation we can incorporate verbal commands that can be understood by the clients. It is also possible to move from visual stimuli to pairing it with verbal command and next moving to verbal commend alone.)

-*Development of passive and "active" vocabulary* (As in the case of verbal commands by introduction of new objects or topics it is possible to extend the vocabulary of our client. We can work both on passive (understanding given word) and also on active (being able to recall the world) vocabulary.)

-*Articulation exercises* (These are exercises that help increase the movement of the mouth, lips, and jaw and improve ability to control speech.)

Inclusion:

EAAT activities most often take place in riding centers that also provide other services to the general population. What's more, a Para-Olympic rider can also participate in main stream dressage competitions. EAAT also provides an opportunity for an activity that the whole family can get involved in at the same time. Some centers provide family lessons and integrated "fun" shows (for example, a Halloween Show).

Now that we have a better understanding of what EAAT is, let's present the scientific proof that it works.

KAROLINA LABRECQUE

RESEARCH ON EAAT

According to I. Strauss (1996, p. 13) the phenomenon of the contact with a horse is a result of a specific relation that includes both the body and the mind. In the therapeutic triangle of the horse-client-therapist, the most important therapeutic role is played by the horse. Utilizing the horse for a therapeutic purpose includes a lot of elements that we are not able to duplicate with any other method. The horse, being the live animal and having ability to move at different gates, and change the tempo and direction can influence the rider on many levels.

In the case of therapy with children that do not walk the horse first and foremost gives the feeling of walking. The children can benefit by the increased ability of locomotion, building up muscle symmetry, preventing contractions and joint immobility. By applying right exercises we can also correct body posture.

Riding a horse also provides vestibular stimulation, improves the work of internal organs, and stimulates senses. The movement provides stimulation of balance and eye sight. The hair in the mane and tail as well as the skin of the horse stimulates the touch. The feel of the animal's temperature and the environment stimulates the hearing and the smell. It is worth mentioning that very often all of these stimuli appear together. For children that are overly sensitive to stimulus it may be too much to handle at the beginning. In such a case it is possible to eliminate some of the stimulus by using proper equipment.

Influence of the horse on social and personal development

There are many publications about the bond between horses and humans and about the benefits of equine assisted activities. Most of these publications, however, are published in popular journals, on the internet, and most are very subjective and very emotionally charged (Splinter-Watkins, 2003). There has been some research done in this field so next we will talk about some of the scientific finding in this field even if it is not directly related to ASD.

The influence of horse on the physical development

Most of the available research in the field of EAAT concentrates on cerebral palsy, which is defined as "a non-progressive, non-contagious motor condition acquired during prenatal development, birth or shortly after birth, that causes physical disability in human development. It exhibits itself chiefly in the various areas of body movement. It is similar to ASD because it is also an umbrella term and as in ASD there are significant neurological changes in the patients. Sometimes the two disorders form dual diagnosis.

Mac Kinnon et al (1995) researched the influence of therapeutic horseback riding on a group of children age 4 to 12. Their quantitative measurements concentrated on the body posture, gross and fine motor control, and daily life skills. The qualitative measurements included observations in the physical, psychological and social progress, and progress in riding skills. The observations where done by the instructor, parents and therapist. Each child also had 3 sessions on the horse recorded. The qualitative analysis showed that the only statistically significant change was present in the case of the fine motor control, but the qualitative analysis showed changes that were not seen during the quantitative analysis. The evaluation of each child by their therapist showed progress in either physical or psychological development and in some cases in both. The biggest progress was noticeable in the body posture, control of the trunk, the mobility of the pelvis, and hand control. There was also improvement in riding skills. The parents observed positive changes in the area of daily life skills, and in the ability to walk. The video analysis also showed positive changes. The children displayed a better position of the head, neck, shoulders, elbows, hips, calves and heels.

Benda et al (2003) researched the influence of hippotherapy on muscular activity of children with CP. The group consisted of 15 children age 4 to 12. A pre and post research model with a control group was utilized. The children were given an EMG test pre and post eight minute hippotherapy sessions in the case the control group on a barrel. The activity of the trunk and upper leg muscles during seating, standing up and walking was measured. Statistically significant improvement in the symmetry of muscle activity in those muscle groups which before session had the biggest asymmetry was noted. There was no statistically significant change after therapy on the barrel.

McGibbon et al (1998) evaluated the influence of an eight week hippotherapy program on energy expenditure during walking (the length, speed and cadence of the step was measured) and on gross motor control (the use of the GMFM test). The research group consisted of five children with spastic cerebral palsy. The pre and posttest model of research was used. After the hippotherapy all five of the children showed significant decrease in the energy expenditure during walking and improvement in the E scale (walking, running, jumping) of GMFM test. The tendency to smaller cadence and lengthening of the straight was also observed.

Hachl et al (1999) used kinematic analysis to research the influence of hippotherapy on two children with cerebral palsy. The research consisted of two parts. In the first part the kinematic analysis of the trunk of the rider and back of the horse was used to describe orientation of posture, stability of posture, and the difference between the movement in the frontal plane of the rider with experience and a person who is just starting horseback riding. Both persons showed two phases of movement due to the influence of the horse. The person with more experience had a more vertical position of the trunk and a delayed reaction to the horse's movement. The second part of research focused on the influence of 12 weeks of weekly hippotherapy sessions on the posture, coordination and functioning of two children. Both children showed two phases of the movement sequence in reaction to the horse movement and also improvement of coordination between upper and lower part of the trunk and between the lower-upper body and the movement of the horse's back.

MaCPhail et al (1998) checked if children with CP had normal balance reactions during horseback riding. Seven healthy children and six children with z CP were videotaped from the back in the frontal plane during horseback riding. The side movement of the trunk of the child and the movement of the horse's back was analyzed. The children with diplegic cerebral palsy showed that 65-75% of the time they had normal balance reactions. The children with quadriplegic cerebral palsy had normal reactions only 10-35% of the time. The authors emphasize that for children with diplegic cerebral palsy it is possible to increase the normal balance reactions through therapy.

Wingate et al (1982) examined the influence of a pilot program on seven clients. The goal was to demonstrate the effectiveness of a riding program on the development of sensory integration and physical fitness. Four of the parents noted improvement in physical fitness of their children. They noticed the improvement of posture, decrease in the number of falls during walking, improvement of sitting posture, increase in the independence of self-care, increase in head control, decrease of spasticity of legs, and improvement when walking.

Besides the research on the influence of hippotherapy on people with CP, there are few other publications about the influence of this method on other disabilities. Winchester et al (2002) researched the influence of a 7 week riding program on the function of gross motor skills and on the speed of walking of seven children age 4 to 7 with different developmental disabilities. The group consisted of two children with CP, two with Down Syndrome, one person with dual diagnosis of Down Syndrome and autism, one with spina bifidia and one with traumatic brain injury. The authors used a pre and posttest method, the Gross Motor Function Measure (GMFM) and the speed of walking on the distance of 10 m. The data analysis showed statistically significant improvement in the results of GMFM. The improvement was also sustained in the repetition of the posttest after 7 weeks from the end of the treatment. There was no statistically significant change in the speed of the walk.

Extensive research on the influence of motor and social development of people with disabilities was also done by Wyżnikiewicz-Nawracała (2002). In her in depth work she described two groups of patients: 33 persons with CP and 35 with other disabilities (Down syndrome, epilepsy, leukemia, Legg-Calvé-Perthes disease, nervosas, and others). The clients participated in therapeutic horseback riding activities for at least 6 month in the center at which the research was conducted. Their age, riding experience, and the length of previous experiences in THR were very diverse. To evaluate improvement in motor development, the author utilized three sets of different exercises. Each case was analyzed separately using descriptive-empirical-analytical method using descriptive categories, points assigned to specific activities, and points for being able to repeat a given exercise in a given time. All of the participants of therapeutic riding achieved improvement in their motor development. The degree and the speed of improvement were precisely described for each client and depended on the type of disability.

Wyżnikiewicz Nawracała (2002) also researched the influence of therapeutic horseback riding on the cognitive, emotional, and social development and of mood. The first three aspects of development were analyzed using the observation of behavior scales from the Weronica Sherborne method. They include descriptive categories. The change in the child's behavior and his or her interaction with the environment were evaluated based on an interview with the parents. All children achieved progress in cognitive, emotional, and social development. Just like in the case of the motor skills, the progress in this case differed in degree and time.

MacKinnon at ell (1995) used two subscales from the Vineland Adaptive Behavior Scale daily living scale (personal skills, home skills, and social skills) and a subscale for socialization which addressed interpersonal relationships, use of leisure time, and stress management. The parents also completed the *Harter Self-Perception Profile,* which allowed researchers to evaluate self-perception of the children of their own school ability, social acceptance, sport abilities, physical appearances, and behavior. Another tool used by the authors to measure social skills, emotional abilities, and behavioral issues was *The Child Behavior Checklist* (CBCL). Parents and therapists were also interviewed. The analyses of the above data did not show statistically significant improvement in any of the scales after the therapeutic horseback riding. Changes were noted by parents and therapists, however. They mostly listed improvements in self-esteem and an increase in social interactions. Parents also mentioned the general improvement in behavior, increase of motivation, higher willingness to experience new things, better self-perception, more willingness to cooperate, and enthusiasm. Also Wingate (1982) noticed (in therapists' observations) improvement in self-perception and happiness from participation in the program.

Resources:

Benda, W., McGibbon, N.H, Grant, K.L. (2003). Improvements in muscle symmetry in children with cerebral palsy after equine-assisted therapy (hippotherapy). *The Journal of Alternative and Complementary Medicine*, 9, 817-825.

Biery M.J. , (1985) Riding and the handicapped. *Vet Clin North Am Small Anim Pract.* 15, p. 345-354.

Clayton, H.M. (2004). *The dynamic horse. A biomechainical guide to equine movement and performance.* Mason, MI: Sport Horse Publications

Grabowski, J. (1982) Hipologia dla wszystkich. Warsaw: Krajowa Agencja Wydawnicza,

Hachl V. et al. (1999) The influence of Hippotherapy on the Kinematics and Functional Performance of Two Children with Cerebral Palsy. *Pediatric Physical Therapy*, 11, 89-101.

Harris, Susan E. ,(1993) *Horse Gait, Balance and Movement* New York: Howell Book House 1993 p. 42-44

http://en.wikipedia.org/wiki/Equestrian_vaulting

http://www.horseshelpingpeoplema.com/eaa.html#efl

http://www.specialolympics.org/.

Łojek J., (2006) Pokrojowe uwarunkowania wyboru konia do hipoterapii. *Przegląd Hipoterapeutyczny.*

MacGibbon N.,H., Andrade C.K., Widener. G. Cintas H.L (1998). Effect of an equine-movement therapy program on gait, energy expenditure, and motor function in children with spastic cerebral palsy: a pilot study. *Developmental Medicine and Child Neurology* 40, 754-762

MacKinon, J., Noh, S., Lariveire, J., MacPhail, A., Allan,.D., (1995) Therapeutic horseback riding: A review of the literature. *Physical & Occupational Therapy in Pediatrics*, 15(1), 1-15.

MacKinon, J., Noh, S., Lariveire, J., MacPhail, A., Allan,.D., i Laliberte, D. (1995) A Study of Therapeutic Effects of Horseback Riding for Children with Cerebral Palsy. *Physical & Occupational Therapy in Pediatrics*, 15(1), 17-31.

MacPhail, H.E, Edwards, J.,G., Miller, K., Mosier, C., Zwiers, T., (1998). Trunk Postural Reaction in Children with and Without Cerebral Palsy During Therapeutic Horseback Riding. *Pediatric Physical Therapy* 10:143-147

Michałowicz. R. red. (1993) Mózgowe porażenie dziecięce. Warszawa: Państwowy Zakład Wydawnictw Lekarskich

Przewloka K., (2007) *Synchronization of Sensory Motor Reactions in Children with Autism during Hippotherapy*. Warsaw: University of Physical Education.

Winchester P., Kendall, K., Peters, H., Sears, N., Winkley, T., (2002). The Effect of Therapeutic Horseback Riding on Gross Motor Function and Gait Speed in Children Who Are Developmentally Delayed. *Physical & Occupational Therapy* in Pediatrics, 22(3/4), 37-50.

Wingate L., (1982). Feasibility of Horseback Riding as a Therapeutic and Integrative Program for Handicapped *Children. Physical Therapy* 62 (2) 184-186.

Wyżnikiewicz Nawracała, A.(2002) *Jeździectwo w rozwoju motorycznym i psychospołecznym osób niepełnosprawnych*. Gdańsk :AWF Gdańsk

PART TWO

AUTISM SPECTRUM DISORDER: THE OVERVIEW

CHAPTER FOUR

WHAT IS AUTISM (BRIEF HISTORY AND DI-AGNOSIS)

Although autism did not formally exist as a separate disorder till 1943 it was previously described under different names. In ancient times doctors qualified it under the label of "God Illnesses". These were serious and unexplainable behavioral disorders (Delacato, 1995). In the 5th Century BC, Herodotus described the story of Krojsos' son who never spoke and was supposedly deaf, but regained his ability to speak as an adult (Brauner, 1993). Early instances of descriptions of autism can also be found in myths and fairy tales. People told stories about small children who were kidnapped or substituted for by bad spirits or witches. Good children (mostly boys) who thus far caused no trouble in life, would suddenly start to behave strangely around the age of two. Their parents mistook this behavior for substitution by a witch and tried to get the "right" child back by different means. Characteristics of autism can be also found in different descriptions of jesters who served in Ancient Rome and in courts of 15th Century aristocracy (Brauner, 1993).

By the end of the 18th Century the approach to people with symptoms on this spectrum changed. Children with autism stopped being treated as miniature adults, who simply require education. We can consider the diaries of Doctor Jean Marc Itard (1801) as one of the first examples of notes about a child with autism. He described the "Savage from Aveyron"[16], a boy who was living in the woods and eating whatever he could find. After he was captured the first time, the child actually ran away. Captured again, he was sent to Paris where he was put into the care of Doctor Itard (Brauner, 1993). Itard de-

---

[16] *An Historical Account of the Discovery and Education of a Savage Man: Or, the First Developments, Physical and Moral, of the Young Savage Caught in the Woods Near Aveyron in the Year 1798* - free full text of the English-language translation of the book; published in 1802 (http://books.google.com/books?id=E63cRcnV2hIC&source=gbs_summary_s&cad=0)

scribed, among others, the following characteristics of the child's behavior: lack of patience, fear, isolation from people, hipoactivity, difficulties with adapting to new situations, lack of personal hygiene,
incorrect functioning of the senses, lack of memory and lack of the
ability to correctly judge situations, lack of attention and problems with
concentration, lack of speech, very high motor abilities, and constant
changes of mood from apathy to over-activity (Zabłocki, 2002).

Another work, possibly a first scientific description of a person
with autism, was "Considerations on the moral management of insane
persons" by Haslam J. (1817, Brauner, 1993). Haslam singled out the
following symptoms: hyperactivity, irritability, lack of the ability focus
on one thing, misbehaving, maniacal behaviors, aggression towards
the immediate environment, vandalism, inability to form relationships
with peers, delay in physical and emotional development, inability to
correctly judge distances, and limited vocabulary.

Kanner (1943) and Asperger (1944) were the first to use the
word "autism". Independently, both men described very similar patients and symptoms. They mentioned problems with social interaction
that the children had and both decided that this is the single most important characteristic of autism. They also both emphasized the difference between autism and childhood schizophrenia. They based they
opinion on three characteristic traits: the lack of hallucinations, improvement of the patients state (as opposed to a decline in health),
and the fact that the children started to show disturbing behaviors very
early in their lives (Happe, F., 1994). Through the years, the description of difficulties with sensory processing, problematic behaviors, and
development of speech are still similar to the one described in the early years of research. Kanner described five key characteristic of autistic child:

1. Lack of an ability to create relationships and bonds
   with people that exists from the beginning of the
   child's life;
2. Inability to communicate with others through speech;
3. Obsessing about changes in the environment, resistance to any changes;
4. Preoccupation with objects rather than people;

5.   Sometimes selective talents in the math, art or music.

Pisula (2002, p. 11) also mentions the five characteristics of autism that were listed by Kanner, but these did not quite withstand the test of time and in some cases were very unfair on the parents or the people with autism. Here are the myths about autism:

1.   Autism as an affect disorder;
2.   Parents of autistic children are "cold" and "overly rational"- the "refrigerator mother" theory;
3.   Autistic children don't have neurological issues.
4.   All autistic children have very high intelligence.
5.   Autistic children come from families with higher socio-economic status.

The theory that autism is caused by parenting was also developed by famous psychoanalyst Bruno Bettelheim. This author claimed that autism is caused by the child's withdrawal from unfriendly and "cold" environment that was created by parents (Landau, 2001). Today we know that this theory is totally untrue and very harmful not only for the parents of people with autism but also for the whole family of people living with autism[17]. So what exactly is autism and what causes it?

Diagnosis

Diagnosis of ASD is not easy. Small children very often do not exhibit homogenous behaviors and characteristics and some of the problems that occur in ASD can be difficult to distinguish from other developmental problems. ASD needs to be differentiated from mental retardation, delay in speech development, attention deficit disorders, problems with learning, and childhood schizophrenia. Problems with sensory integration, which will be discuss in much more detail later in this book, although very characteristic for autism, can also be present in other disorders.

---

[17] If you would like to learn more about 70 years of diagnosis of autism you can go here: http://www.nejm.org/doi/full/10.1056/NEJMp1306380.

As the theories about the roots of autism changed, so did the model of viewing this disorder. At the beginning, as it was in the case of Kanner's theory, autism was considered a disease. The next attempt of classification was the proposition of Christopher Gilberg (1992) to treat autism as a subtype of a broader category of affect disorders. Today we view autism as a spectrum (Autism Spectrum Disorder, ASD), which encompasses (according to Wing, 1997, Pislula, 2002) "all people which show even smallest of symptoms from the triad of problems in:

1. Social interactions;
2. Verbal and nonverbal communication;
3. Imagination (repetitive/stereotypic behaviors)."

Currently the most common way of diagnosing autism is using the criteria of Diagnostic and Statistical Manual (DSM). DSM IV used to lists five Pervasive Developmental Disorders (PDDs), commonly known as Autism Spectrum Disorders (ASDs). They were:

1. Autistic Disorder
2. Pervasive Developmental Disorder, Not Otherwise Specified
3. Asperger's Disorder
4. Rett Disorder
5. Childhood Disintegrative Disorder

However in the new edition of DSM -DSMV Pervasive Developmental Disorders disappeared and in their place two new categories of autism spectrum disorder (ASD) and related diagnosis of social communication disorders were created. Here are the new criteria for ASD diagnosis:

A. Persistent deficits in social communication and social interaction across multiple contexts, as manifested by the following, currently or by history:
    1. Deficits in social- emotional reciprocity, ranging, for example, from abnormal social approach and failure of normal back-and –forth conversation; to reduced

sharing of interests, emotions, or affect; to failure to initiate or respond to social interactions.

2. Deficits in nonverbal communicative behaviors used for social interaction, ranging, for example, from poorly integrated verbal and nonverbal communication; to abnormalities in eye contact and body language or deficits in understanding and use of gestures; to a total lack of facial expressions and nonverbal communication.

3. Deficits in developing, maintaining, and understanding relationships, ranging, for example, from difficulties adjusting behavior to suit various social context; to difficulties in sharing imaginative play or in making friends; to absence of interest in peers.

B. Restricted, repetitive patterns of behavior, interests or activities, as manifested by at least two of the following, currently or by history.

1. Stereotyped or repetitive motor movements, use of objects, or speech (e.g., simple motor stereotypes, lining up toys or flipping objects, echolalia, idiosyncratic phrases).

2. Insistence on sameness, inflexible adherence to routines, or ritualized patterns or verbal nonverbal behavior (e.g., extreme distress at small changes, difficulties with transitions, rigid thinking patterns, greeting rituals, need to take a same route or eat same food every day).

3. Highly restricted, fixated interests that are abnormal in intensity or focus (e.g., strong attachment to or preoccupation with unusual objects, excessively circumscribed or preservative interest).

4. Hyper –or hyporeactivity to sensory input or unusual interests in sensory aspects of the environment (e.g., apparent indifference to pain/temperature, adverse response to specific sounds or textures, excessive smelling or touching of objects, visual fascination with lights or movement).

The criteria require to specify current severity, which is based on social communication impairments and restricted, repetitive patterns of behavior[18].

C. Symptoms must be present in the early developmental period (but may not become fully manifest until social demands exceed limited capacities, or may be masked by learned strategies in later life).
D. Symptoms cause clinically significant impairment in social, occupational, or other important areas of current functioning.
E. These disturbances are not better explained by intellectual disability (intellectual developmental disorder) or global developmental delay. Intellectual disability and autism spectrum disorder frequently co-occur; to make comorbid diagnosis of autism spectrum disorder and intellectual disability; social communication should be below that expected for general developmental level.

Since now we know what is currently considered ASD, we can move on to the next, very important and controversial topic: the etiology of autism.

Etiology of autism

As mentioned previously, the first theory about etiology of autism was based on the assumption that there is a deficit in the child-parent interaction. Currently researchers agree that autism is not a psychological disorder and it has an organic basis.

The causes of autism and theories about them are as different as each child. So far no one has been able to pin point a single factor that can cause ASD. Researchers are concentrating on the genetic and environmental factors. While the debate continues, they all agree that ASD has neurobiological origins. The topic of the etiology of au-

---

[18] For the specific description of three levels of severity (requiring support, requiring substantial support and requiring very substantial support) and full criteria of ASD please visit:
http://depts.washington.edu/dbpeds/Screening%20Tools/DSM-5(ASD.Guidelines)Feb2013.pdf

tism is too extensive to be discussed in much detail in this book. If you are interested to find out more about current research on autism please refer to the Resources part of this chapter. Below is a simple explanation of the neuropsychological bases of autism that are relevant to EAAT. If you are not interested in learning about different brain structures and the medical terminology, please skip straight to the next chapter.

Neurobiology of autism

In his work, Delacato (1995) discussed the causes of autism proposing that they are based on brain damage. He noticed discrete neurological problems in children with autism: weak coordination, delays in development, squinting, problems with lateralization, tip toeing, problems with balance, problems with reflexes, hyperactivity, weak manual skills, disorderly sensory reception, problems with concentration, and significant problems with learning. According to Delacato people with autism attempt to use the damaged sensory channels, that lead from the receptors to the brain through their (either aggressive or stereotypic) behavior.

Current literature (Courchesne, et al., 1994; Balley et al, 1996; Pisula, 2002; Huebner, 2001; Wong 1991; Rapin and Katzman, 1998, and others) mentions four main structures of the central nervous system that may be causing problems: the brain stem, cerebellum, medial temporal lobes, and the areas of the brain which are responsible for cognitive and executive functions.

Cerebellum

The cerebellum is the region of the brain which plays an important role in motor control. It is also involved in some cognitive functions such as attention and language, and probably in some emotional functions such as regulating fear and pleasure responses[19]. Among its complete list of functions we can find:

- Posture and balance control;

---

[19] Wolf U, Rapoport MJ, Schweizer TA (2009). "Evaluating the affective component of the cerebellar cognitive affective syndrome". *J. Neuropsychiatry Clin. Neurosci.* **21** (3): 245–53.

- Muscle tone control;
- Coordination of willful movement;
- Modulation of sensory stimulation;
- Integration of sensory stimulation in the brain;
- Sequencing;
- Development of speech;
- Nonverbal communication;
- Concentration.

The cerebellum is built from, among other things, Purkinje cells, which receive information from the eyes, touch, prioprioception, balance and hearing. Research has showed (Bauman and Kemper, 1994: Courchesne et al., 1994; Rapin and Katmzna, 1998) that in autistic people there is a significant decrease in the number of these cells. Gliman, S. Newman, S.W. (1992) mention that problems within the brain stem can lead to lower muscle tone, lower ability for coordination, inappropriate feeling of time, slow, monotonous speech, lower ability and problems with sensory modulation. Other sources (Jones and Prior, 1985; Kemmer et al, 1998; Kohen-Raz, Volkmar and Cohen 1992) also point to significant motor problems in people with autism. Some authors (Harbert, M.R. 2002; Schmahamann, 1994) draw attention to other functions of the cerebellum (processing of emotions and social situations, nonverbal communication, regulation of the speed of thoughts and appropriate time reactions) with which people with autism often have problems.

Brain Stem

The brain stem, though small, is an extremely important part of the brain as the nerve connections of the motor and sensory systems from the main part of the brain to the rest of the body pass through it. The brain stem includes a lot of the nuclei that are associated with processing of the sensory and motor impulses (including nuclei of ten out of the twelve cranial nerves), and tracts for motor, the fine touch, vibration sensation and prioprioception, pain, temperature, itch and crude touch. The brain stem also plays an important role in the regulation of the cardiac and respiratory functions. It regulates the central nervous system, and is pivotal in maintaining consciousness and regulating the sleep cycle.

People with autism have a lot of paradoxical symptoms as far as concentration goes. For example they can be less sensitive to pain and more sensitive to other stimuli. They can have a very high ability to concentrate on activities which they initiated and at the same time a very short attention span for activities that have a social context or which they are not interesting in for themselves. Often we can see over-reactivity to one type of stimuli (sound or smell, for instance) and under-sensitivity to another (ex. touch). Autistic people often have trouble sleeping as well (Huebner and Lane, 2001). Stereotypical movements and self-mutilation are often interpreted as an attempt at compensation for modulation of stimuli and of keeping the homeostasis in the overly stimulated or under stimulated environment (Berkson, 1996; Guess and Carr, 1991). In their work Huebner and Lane (2001) mentioned that at the beginning of their research they concentrated on the brain stem because that's where the problems with sensory processing are most often localized.

The brain stem is a part of the Social Engagement System (Porges, 2006). This is a model which explains how neurological structures are engaged in social behaviors and emotions. "Social communication depends on cortical regulation of medullar nuclei via corticobulbar pathways. The social engagement system consists of a somatomotor component (special visceral efferent pathways that regulate the muscles of the head and face) and a visceromotor component (the myelinated vagus that regulates the heard and bronchi). (Portges, 2006, p 70).

We can also associate problems with vagus nerve with the brain steam. As mentioned above, among other things it is an important component of the social engagements system. It also regulates the heart rate and heart rate variability as well as the work of the intestines. The stimulation of this nerve has proven effective in the treatment of depression and epilepsy. Although so far no one is using the direct stimulation of this nerve in the treatment of autism, Porges (2006) suggests the possibility of indirect stimulation through peripheral baroreceptors that regulate blood pressure. "Rocking and swinging, in which the position of the head is changed relative to the position of the heart, will stimulate the baroreceptors and engage feedback loop. This suggests that the frequently observed rocking and swinging behaviors in autistic individuals may reflect a naturally occurring bio-behavioral strategy to stimulate and regulate a vagal system that is not efficiently functioning." (Porgers 2006, p. 73)

Medial temporal lobe and surrounding areas

Medial temporal lobes are responsible for perception of hearing, integration of visual stimulus with all other sensory information, and for reception of olfactory stimuli. A part of the medial temporal lobe is also included in the limbic system, which is responsible mostly for emotions, but also for aggression, defense mechanisms, and reactions to pain and regulation of the process of sleep and arousal. The limbic system includes the hippocampus, amygdala, anterior thalamic nuclei, septum, limbic cortex and fornix.

Waterhouse et al (1996) after reviewing the literature list four main dysfunctional areas in medial temporal lobes, which may cause autism. The first area is associated with increased density and decrease in size of the cells in the hippocampus[20]. This brain structure is mostly responsible for memory (recent memory) and plays a major role in the learning process, representational or declarative memory, and procedural memory. This last one, procedural memory, appears to be intact in people with autism since they often demonstrate stronger visual perceptual memory. The hippocampus also helps filter sensory input from the environment. This process allows avoiding sensory overstimulation. Problems within the hippocampus lead to inappropriate sensory integration and to difficulties in changing attention between different stimuli. They also lead to smaller amounts of available working memory, which is necessary for carrying a conversation and for symbolic play.[21]

The second dysfunctional area is associated with undervaluing a giving sensory or social stimulus. This problem is connected with increased density and a decrease in size of the cells in the amygdale. This structure plays a major role in deciding if the given stimulus is linked with danger and in basic emotional reactions[22]. This nucleus

---

[20] (Huebner, and Lane 2001; Bauman, 2006).
[21] (Huebner and Lane, 2001).
[22] (Ledoux, 1996).

also plays a role in attaching an emotional meaning to a given stimulus (for example: facial expression, gesture, punishment, reward, etc.). Problems within this area cause difficulties with regard to emotions, with facial recognition, with memory, and with recognizing emotional context. They can also lead to lower social activity and problems with behaviors associated with communication[23].

The third dysfunctional area according to Waterhouse et al. (1996) is being asocial. The researchers think that this state can be associated with abnormal levels of neuropeptides: oxytocin and vasopressin[24]. They are synthesized in the hypothalamus and released by the pituitary gland. The receptors for this substance are located in the structures of the temporal lobe and thalamus, in the limbic system, and in parts of the brain stem. They are also a part of the social engagement system described earlier. Oxytocin is considered a substance which promotes expression of behaviors that are necessary for forming and keeping social relations[25].

Waterhouse et al. (1996) proposed that the forth primary dysfunctional area of deficits in autism is extended selective attention. This problem arises due to incorrect development in the parietal and temporal polysensory association areas. Hass et al. (1996) showed through MRI that people with autism have smaller parietal lobes and smaller corpus callosum. Damage in this area leads to the narrowing of selective attention to single aspects of sensory stimuli. In the case of people with autism it can be a tremendous problem (oversensitivity or undersensitivity, concentration on only one stimulus, inability to synchronize stimuli), but it may also lead to outstanding ability in the areas of visual or auditory processing.

Cognitive executive functions

The areas of the brain responsible for cognitive and executive functions are also taken under consideration in the etiology of autism. Cognitive functions such as planning, voluntary eye gaze, spontaneity, metacognition, and response inhibition and judgment in social and

---

[23] (Huebner and Lane, 2001)

[24] (Huebner and Lane, 2001).

[25] (Huebner and Kreamer, 2001)

sexual behavior are associated with frontal lobes (Huebner and Lane 2001). Some researchers (Clark and Plante, 1998; Leonard et al., 1996; Herbert et al., 2002; De Fosse et al., 2002) are proving that autistic people who have major problems with speech and communication have an asymmetry of the left hemisphere in comparison to neuro-typical people. This work is counterbalanced, however, by other researchers (Dunn., M, 1994; Piven & O'Leary, 1997) through publications that show no asymmetry in the frontal lobe. Further research is need in this area.

Influence of movement on the brain

There is one more aspect of neuropsychology that I think is worth mentioning since it may shed some light understanding why EAAT may have such a positive influence on the autistic population. That aspect is the influence of movement on the brain and brain development.

In order to make any kind of movement we need to coordinate sensory information coming from the environment with priopriocep-tion[26] and with the ability to execute movement. Szop (1996) mentions that we all have motor predispositions, which can be divided into structural, energetic, coordination, and psychological. In this chapter I would like to concentrate on the coordination predispositions since they refer to the "ability of the organism to make precise movement in a changing environment" (Szop et al., 1996, p. 38). The bases of these predispositions lay in the neuro-physiological mechanisms of movement control located on different levels of the central nervous system. Raczek et al. (2003) proposed a simplified scheme showing the structures of the central nervous system and their connections and the role that they play in the regulation of movement[27]. This scheme includes four areas of the brain that, in case of people with autism, are often not working properly. The scheme also shows an important role played by sensory receptors which are also not working properly in the ASD population. At different stages of the motor program (plan-

---

[26] Prioprioception-ability to receive stimuli from within the organism (eg through muscles, tendons and joints) – The New Lexicon Webster's Dictionary of the English Language 1989

[27] If you are interested to learn more about this process please visit www.thehealinghorses.com/ movement?

ning, programming, execution, correction) different levels of the central nervous system are activated (Szop et al., 1996, Raczek et al., 2003). Planning and optimization happen in the subcortical motivational pathways and in the association cortex. From here the motor programs are sent to effectors through two systems: the pyramidal track or the extrapyramidal system. The pyramidal track is responsible for controlling complex voluntary movements and posture. It includes motor areas which consist of corticospinal track and cortico-motoneural track. They transfer the signals to the spinal cord and branch out to many subcortical structures (basal ganglia, cerebellum, etc) and receive signals from priprioreceptors and from some of the receptors for hearing and sight. The extrapyramidal system is responsible for automatic or semi automatic movements. It receives information about the current environmental status and motor system. So it controls movement and muscle tone. It influences motor activity associated with posture and reflexes. It works through the thalamus, motor cortex, and the corticobulbar and corticospinal systems (Fix, 1997). These systems cooperate with the pyramidal track and are located on all the levels of the central nervous system.

The next level of control over coordination is created by the basal ganglia and cerebellum. Basal ganglia (which also include the previously described amygdale) direct attention to a new stimulus and control the effectiveness of learned motor activity. They are also a part of the limbic system. The cerebellum is a part of the pyramidal system and the extra-pyramidal system. It controls most human movement. It takes part in creation of all motor programs both on the level of learning a new program and on the level of correcting the existing program (Szopa et al., 1996 Raczek et al., 2003).

Based on the neurophysiology of the mechanism of control, Szopa et al. (1996) proposes two categories of coordination predispositions:

1. Predispositions based on the ability to engage already existing motor programs. It could be done through sensory stimuli or through direct command from the motor cortex. The authors include in this category:

a. The reaction time (simple and complex) to a different stimuli (visual, audio, tactile);
b. Coordination between the receptors and movement (visual-audio-tactile);
c. Speed-frequency of movement (the agility of the processes of stimulation and inhibition);
d. Prioprioception;
e. Differentiation between the movements (complex function of proprioceptors and control centers);
f. Rhythm of movements (it involves the function of motor and tactical centers);
g. Balance (a complex function of system of prioprioceptors, vestibule, and control centers).

2. Predispositions that matter during creation of new motor programs, also known as motor skills. They are based on the network of feedback between receptors and control centers and between feedback from the neural network crated in the process of learning new movements or correction of the movements that has been already learned. Motor skills include: the speed of learning, the precision of learning, and the permanence of learning.

The research showed (Raczek et al., 2003) that a different coordination exercise done by a group of neurotypical children had a positive effect not only on the development of different coordination and motor behaviors, but also on the function of perception, sensor-motor reaction, memory, intellectual activity, and on functions that promote correct control processes and regulation of motor activities.

Children with ASD often have problems with sensory integration and with motor control. The development of neuro-rehabilitation in the 1950's led to the creation of different therapeutic approaches characterized by different underlining theories (Kwolek, 2003). Two of them were the NDT-Bobath and sensory integration (which is described later in this book on page 71). Both of these therapeutic methods were influenced by the work of Margaret Rood (Rydeen K., 2001). She emphasized three therapeutic principals that where later crucial for the development of the two therapies mentioned above:

1. Controlled sensory stimulation
2. Use of developmental sequencing
3. The need to require and facilitate a purposeful response through the use of activity (Rydeen, 2001).

According to Bobath[28] the normal motor development of humans is the result of:

- Undisturbed integration of the brain function in the process of accommodation of the body to the environment.
- Correct development of the mechanism of postural control do to correct muscle tone, organization of nervous system, correct coordination of postural and motor control.
- Variability of the motor development do to the maturation of CNS and due to the improvement of the motor response to the stimuli from the sensory learning;
- Developmental, memory, and corrective plasticity due to the permanent functional changes in response to given sensory stimuli, giving the chance for development and correction of some disorders in the immature CNS (Kwolek, 2003 p 403).

Learning motor functions that can later be used in daily living skills is conditioned by senso- motor experiences (Kwolek, 2003). Rydeen (2001) described a sensory-motor-sensory loop which can be influenced both by sensory integration therapy and by NDT intervention. The brain registers incoming sensory stimuli, which are then interpreted and influence the motor reaction, which in turn provides new sensory stimulus. The NDT works on the motor reaction side of the loop while the sensory integration works through manipulation of sensory input. More about that will be said in the next chapter which will focus

---

[28] The Bobath concept is named after its inventors: Berta Bobath (physiotherapist) and Karel Bobath (a psychiatrist/neurophysiologist). Their work focused mainly on patients with cerebral palsy and stroke. The main problems of these patient groups resulted in a loss of the normal postural reflex mechanism and normal movements.[5] At its earliest inception, the Bobath concept was focused on regaining normal movements through re-education. Since then, it has evolved to incorporate new information on neuroplasticity, motor learning and motor control. (http://en.wikipedia.org/wiki/Bobath_concept).

on different therapeutic modalities in autism and how EAAT can be integrated within each.

Resources

Bauman, M.,L., Kemper, T., I. (1994) Neuroanatomical observations of the brain in autism. In: Bauman, M., L. Kemper T., L. red (2006) *The Neurobiology of Autism.* The Johns Hopkins University Press: Baltimore.

Berkson, (1996). Feedback and control in the development of abnormal stereotyped behaviors. In R. Sprague & K. Newell (Eds.) *Stereotyped movements: Brain and behavior relationships* (pp. 3-15). Washington, DC: APA.

Brauner A. F.,(1993). *Dziecko zagubione w rzeczywistości.* Wydawnictwa Szkolne i Pedagogiczne, Warszawa

Clark M., Plante E. (1998) Morphology of the inferior frontal gyrus in developmentally language disordered adults. *Brain Language* 61: 288-303

Courchesne, E., Townsend J., Saitoh O. (1994). The brain in infantile autism: Posterior fossa structures are abnormal. *Neurology* 44: 214-223.

De Fosse, Hodge S., Harris G, et al. (2002). An abnormal volumetric asymmetry pattern in language processing cortical areas in children with autism and children with SLI. *Presented at the conference: International Meeting for Autism Research*, Orlando, Fla., November 1-2

Delacato C. H., (1995) *Dziwne, niepojętne.* Autystyczne Dziecko. Fundacja Synapsis, Warszawa

Dunn W. (1994) Performance of Typical Children on the Sensory Profile: An Item Analysis. *The American Journal of Occupational Therapy* 48 (11)" 967-974

Fix J. (1997) *Neuroanatomia*. Urban & Partner. Wydawnictwo Medyczne Wrocław.

Gillberg C. (1992) Subgroups in autism: are there behavioural phenotypes typical of underlying medical conditions? *J Intell Disab Res* 36:201-14.

Gliman, S. Newman, S.W. (1992) *Essentials of Clinical Neuroanatomy and Neurophysiology (8ed)* Philadelphia: F.A. Davis.

Guess, D., & Carr, E. (1991). Emergence and maintenance of stereotypy and self-injury. *American Journal on Mental Retardation*, 96, 299-319

Happe, F., (1994). *Autism: an introduction to psychological theory*. Harvard University Press, Cambridge Massachusetts.

Hass, R. H., Townsend, J. Courchesne, E., Lincoln,. A. J., Schreibman, L., i Yeung-Courchesne R. (1996) Neurological abnormalities in infantile autism. *Journal of Child Neurology*, 11, 84-92.

Herbert MR, Harris GJ, Adrien Kt, et al. (2002). Abnormal asymmetry in language association cortex in autism. *Annals of Neurology* 52: 588-96.

Herbert MR, Harris GJ, Adrien Kt, et al. (2002). Abnormal asymmetry in language association cortex in autism. *Annals of Neurology* 52: 588-96.

Huebner i Lane (2001). Neuropsychological Findings, Etiology, and Implications for Autism. W: Huebner, R. (2001). Autism: a sensory motor approach. Maryland: Aspen Publishers' Inc.

Jones V., Prior M. (1985). Motor Imitation Abilities and Neurological Signs in Autistic Children. Journal of Autism and Developmental Disorders, 5: 37-45.

Kemner C. , C., Verbaten, M. N., Cuperus, J. M., Camfferman, G. & van Engeland, H (1998). Abnormal Saccadic Eye Movements in Autistic Children. Journal of Autism and Developmental Disorders 28(1): 61-67

Kohen-Raz R., Volkmar F, R., Cohen D. J (1992) Postural Control in Children with Autism. *Journal of Autism and Developmental Disorders* 22(3): 419-432

Kwolek, A. Ed. (2003). *Rehabilitacja medyczna Tom II.* Wydawnictwo Medyczne Urban & Partner. Wrocław.

Landau, E., (2001). *Autism.* Franklin Watts, NY

Leonard C., Lombardino L., Mercado L, et al. (1996) Cerebral asymmetry and cognitive development in children: a magnetic resonance imaging study. *Psychological Science* 7: 79-85.

Neuro-Developmental Treatment (NDT) http://www.ndta.org/

Pisula E., (2002). *Autyzm u dzieci. Diagnoza, klasyfikacje etiologia.* Wydawnictwo Naukowe PWN, Warszawa

Piven & O'Leary, D. (1997). Neuroimaging in autism. *Children and Adolescence Psychiatric Clinics of North America*, 6, 305-323.

Porges, S. (2006). The Vagus: A Mediator of Behavioral and Physiologic Features Associated with Autism. W: Bauman, M., L. I Kemper T., L. red (2006) *The Neurobiology of Autism.* The Johns Hopkins University Press: Baltiomore.

Raczek J., Młynarski W., Liach W. (2003) *Kształtowanie i diagnozowanie koordynacyjnych zdolności motorycznych.* AWF Kraków.

Rapi I., Katzman R. (1998) Neurobiology of Autism. *Annals of Neruology* Vol 43: 7-14.

Rydeen K., (2001) Integration of Sensorimotor and Neurodevelopmental Approches. In: Huebner, R. (2001). *Autism: a sensory motor approach.* (pp.247-261)Maryland: Aspen Publishers' Inc.

Schmahmann, J.D. (1994). The cerebellum in autism: Clinical and anatomical perspectives. In . In: Bauman, M., L. Kemper T., L. (Eds)).*The Neurobiology of Autism.* (pp. 195-226). Baltimore: The Johns Hopkins University Press.

KAROLINA LABRECQUE

Szopa, J., Mleczko E., żak S. (1996) *Podstawy Antropomotoryki*. PWN Warszawa –Kraków 1996.

Waterhouse, L., Fein, D., Modahl, C. (1996) Neurofunctional mechanisms in autism. *Psychological Review,* 103, 457-489.

Zabłocki, K.J (2002) *Autyzm*. Wydawnictwo Naukowe Novum, Płock

PART THREE

MOST COMMON THERAPEUTIC AP-PROACHES IN AUTISM AND HOW THE HORSE CAN BE UTILIZE WITHIN EACH

"If there is anything that we wish to change in the child, we should first examine it and see whether it is not something that could better be changed in ourselves."

– C.G. Jung

The complexity and heterogeneity of autism spectrum disorders lead to the formation of different therapeutic methods. In this chapter I would like to concentrate on the most common current therapeutic methods and also on methods that utilize movement, since those are the most pertinent to the EAATs. In the following chapter I will also discuss how EAAT can be used within a different therapeutic modality and how practitioners of EAAT can benefit from each method. First on the list is a modality that can be integrated with many other therapies and one in which EAAT may play a big role: sensory integration.

CHAPTER FIVE

Sensory Integration

Sensory integration is the "ability to organize the input from multiple senses for use in adaptive response." (Hubner 2001 p.13). It involves the input from all systems of the body (muscle, joints, skin, vestibular receptors, eyes, hearing, etc). According to different authors (Bobkowicz-Lewartowska, 2005, Delecato, Rydeen, 2001 and others) sensory integration should form the basis of all therapy for people with ASD since it prepares the grounds for development and further work. It shows better results if paired with (Rydeen, 2001, Szot, 2004) some kind of movement therapy (ex. earlier mentioned NDT, Shot's method, V. Sherbone's method).

The first propagator of sensory integration was Jean Ayres. Her approach is based on understanding the relation between the brain and behavior and the understanding of neuroscience (Fisher and Murray, 1991). According to the theory of sensory integration the sensory system is based on three basic senses: balance, touch, and prioprioception. Together with sight and hearing these are considered fundamental for the development of more complex functions. Sight and hearing are based on the first three senses (Rydeen, 2001).

All five senses form the first level of sensory integration (Rydeen, 2001)[29] called the primary sensory system. The sub-cortical processes of sensory information coming from these three basic systems are the foundation for development and learning processes. When they cooperate with hearing and vision they function properly. This is possible through the central nervous system (CNS) which registers, interprets, and organizes incoming information. As a result, the organism can develop new skills (Rydeen, 2001). The first level of

---

[29] The four levels of sensory integration had been described in C.S. Kranowitz, The Out-Of-Sync Child, p. 48. Skylight Press Book, 1998

sensory integration is usually complete by the second month of a child's life.

Receptors of the vestibular sense are located in the inner ear and react to gravitation and movement. Its neural connections are spread all over the CNS. Stimulus from this system influences the control of eye balls, level of arousal, emotional reactions, and muscle tone (Rydeen, 2001). Oversensitivity of this system causes the child to avoid movement. The under-sensitivity can lead to hyperactivity. The vestibular system is one form of prioprioception.

Prioprioception according to Stedman's Medical Dictionary[30] is "a sense or perception, usually at a subconscious level, of the movements and positions of the body and especially its limbs, independent of vision; this sense is gained primarily from input from sensory nerve terminals in muscle and tendons and the fibrous capsule of joints combined with input from the vestibular apparatus." This system can be stimulated through movement or through resistance and friction. During those movements the joints are slightly pressed together or stretched. The information about the range of movement and force is then sent to the brain (Dunn and Donaldson, 2001). The vestibular system provides the information about spatial positioning of our body and tells us where our limbs are. Both systems create a reference point for movement control (Rydeen, 2001).

Touch (the tactile system) in the theory of sensory integration can be divided into two separate systems (Rydeen, 2001; Dunn and Donaldson, 2001): discriminative and protective. The protective system informs us, for example, about a spider crawling on our skin. The discriminative system allows us to remove an object from our pocket without looking at it. Both systems give information about our outside environment, but development of the discriminative system contributes to development of skills. Oversensitivity to touch can lead children to avoid physical contact, to an obsessive need to keep their hands clean, to problems with dressing and keeping clothes on, and to very specific ways of shaking hands (tips of the fingers – minimalization of the surface that's being touched). According to

[30] Stedmans's Medical Dictionary 26th Edition, Willams & Wilkins 1995.

Bobkowicz-Lewartoswka (2005) an oversensitivity to touch can be decreased by delivering deep pressure stimulus which activates prioprioception. Conversely, under-sensitivity to touch can be exhibited through injuring a given part of body (ex. biting the hand, hitting the head against a wall). Different, safe forms of stimulation of the affected areas can lead to decrease of undesired behaviors.

The second level of sensory integration is usually complete by the end of the first year of life and forms the perceptual motor foundation. It consists of motor planning (praxis), lateralization (hand preference), bilateral coordination (ability to use both sides of the body in synchronization), and body awareness. This is followed by the development of perceptual motor skills, which is usually completed by the age 3. During this phase the child adds to its skill set many purposeful activities, visual motor integration, hand-eye coordination (pencil skills), and visual and auditory perception. The last, fourth stage of sensory integration developments is academic readiness. Most children reach this level by the age of six. It includes self-esteem and self-control, visualization, specialization of body and brain, organized behavior, regulation of attention, complex motor skills, and academic skills. The levels of sensory integration are sequential and form a pyramid. The correct development of higher skills is impossible without first acquiring the lower level skills.

Sensory Integration and EAAT

The two primary ways of applying the principals of sensory integration through EAAT would be hippotherapy and therapeutic horseback riding. In both situations seating on the horse provides vestibular stimulation. The skin, saddle, saddle pad, and mane all provide different levels of tactical stimulation and different temperature. The use of different toys, therapeutic equipment, and horse brushes can also provide different sources for the tactical experience. The sounds from the surroundings and hoof beats stimulate the auditory sense.

As I mention in Part One of this book, the instructor can influence the stimulation through horse movement by choosing a specific horse, or by changing the position of the client on the horse. There are three basic positions that pertain to SI: calming, stimulation, and neutral. It is very important to remember that a position which may be calming for one client may also be stimulating or neutral for a different client and vice versa. It all depends on the previously mentioned sensory needs. For example a client who seeks vestibular and prioprioceptive stimulation may exhibit hyperactivity and a tendency to seek extreme stimulus (ex. falling from a horse on purpose). Placing such a client prone position over the horse's barrel provides both extensive vestibular and proproceptive stimulation and can help to calm him or her. A similar effect can be achieved by choosing a prone position on the horse's back (lying on the horses back while facing the tail) or supine position (lying on the horses back while facing forward). The same positions used in the case of a client with high sensitivity to stimulus may cause overstimulation and lead to shut down, agitation, or aggressive behaviors.

Another way in which the therapist can manipulate the level of stimulation is the choice of horse. By picking a horse with a short, bouncy step or small barrel we can provide more stimulation. A horse that has a smooth long straight and is wider and not too bouncy can be use for clients who don't need much stimulation. Sometimes we may want to slowly get the client used to stimuli that initially prove to be quite a challenge. This way the brain has a chance to form new connections and acquire new experiences. The range of stimuli that the client can deal with is being expended and can be carried over to everyday situations. In order to do so we may slowly introduce new exercises or a new level of stimulation. For example instead of switching the client to a horse that naturally provides more stimuli, the instructor may first introduce a faster pace at walk or try the trot. He or she can also work on serpentines, and later progress to more sharp turns. The positions on the horse can also be gradually changed to more demanding ones and the time that the client spends in each can be slowly increased.

As I mentioned before, sensory integration can be used in combination with different therapeutic methods. The same cannot be said about combining different therapeutic approaches. It is important that instructors, parents, and the therapist communicate about which modality they are working with, since some approaches to autism utilize totally different and opposite principles. Below is a short introduction to the most popular therapies and the ways that EAAT can supplement them.

Resources:

Bobkowicz-Lewartowska, L. (2005). Autyzm dziecięcy: zagadnienia diagnoza i terapia. Oficyna Wydawnicza Impuls, Kraków.

Delacato C. H., (1995) Dziwne, niepojętne. Autystyczne Dziecko. Fundacja Synapsis, WarszaSzot, Z (2004). Autyzm – terapia ruchowa badania interdyscyplinarne. AWF Gdańsk.

Dunn L.S., Donaldson C. (2001). Integration of the Sensorimotor Approach within the Classroom. W : Huebner, R. (2001). Autism: a sensory motor approach. S:297-311 Maryland: Aspen Publishers' Inc.

Fisher A.G., Murray, E.A. (1991) Introduction to sensory integration theory. In Fisher A.G. Murray, E. A., Bundy A.C. (red.). Sensoryintegration theory and practice (s. 3-26). Filadelfia :F.A. Davis.

Huebner, R.A., Dunn, W., (2001) Introduction and Basic Concepts. W: Huebner, R. (2001). Autism: a sensory motor approach. Maryland: Aspen Publishers' Inc.

CHAPTER SIX

Applied Behavioral Analysis. (ABA)

First developed by Psychologist Ivar Lovaas at the Lovaas Institute for Early Intervention at UCLA, ABA is currently one of the most popular interventions and a base for many educational programs. It focuses on teaching and reinforcing appropriate behaviors and eliminating the inappropriate ones.

ABA is based on the concept of behavior analysis, which is a scientific approach to understanding behavior and how it is affected by the environment. One of the most important concepts in behavior analysis is operant conditioning. This is the idea that one can use external reinforcement to increase the likelihood of a particular behavior occurring. Children with ASD very often have problems with learning from their environment. External rewards can act as motivators and increase the motivation of the child to learn and try new things.

The ABA analyzes three dimensions of the behavior[31]:

> - *Antecedents of behavior.* Analyzing what happened before behavior occurred, the surroundings, different stimulus etc., helps in discovering what caused a given behavior. If we know why someone behaves the way they do, we can predict and eliminate or reinforce a given behavior. This technique is useful no matter what treatment or approach one uses.

> - *Behavior itself:* What role does it play? What meaning does it have?

---

[31] "Behavior" refers to all kinds of actions and skills (not just misbehavior) and "environment" includes all sorts of physical and social events that might change or be changed by one's behavior.

> ➤ *Consequence of behavior.* What happens after a behavior occurs? Does the environment support the given behavior? Does the child get something desirable out of acting the way it is in a given moment?

In addition to analyzing a given behavior, ABA utilizes another tool that can be very useful in many situations, the *discrete trial method*. The discrete trial method was the very first method used within ABA. It utilizes the idea of analyzing a task or routine and breaking it into parts which are manageable and teachable. Subsequently each part is taught separately and finally all of them are chained together. This method takes place in a one-on-one setting. If the child does the task correctly a reward is provided. No reinforcement is given for incorrect response. As good as this method sounds it has one big down side. Life is full of surprises. Utilizing this method seldom leads to generalization. If one of the steps needs sudden adjustment or a task requires an extra step that was not initially practiced, the child may have problems with executing the whole chain in real life. However, this technique is very good when introducing new exercise or new situations and can be helpful for children who cannot function outside a very structured and routine environment.

It is worth mentioning that ABA has evolved through the years and currently the emphasis is placed on engaging the child on its own terms. Strictly sitting at the table and repeating a given task routine has shifted to learning in natural settings. The lessons are structured in a way that encourages the use of the child's own curiosity about a subject. The process resembles the natural learning process of children rather than a rigid classroom exercise or skills training. The emphasis on praise and reinforcement of behavior that parents want their child to engage in is second nature to most parents. Positive reinforcements encourage the neurotypical child to practice and expand their skills. By formalizing this naturally occurring phenomenon ABA minimizes the distractions and sensory input that a child with ASD can find difficult to handle. Many people with ASD do well in a very structured, routine environment and ABA provides that.

KAROLINA LABRECQUE

Application of ABA in EAAT.

EAAT can be easily integrated within the ABA frame work. A lot of techniques used with ABA are also utilized in EAAT's. The new skills are very often taught through the discreet trail method and the lessons are very structured. A lot of EAAT are set up in one-on-one setting or even one client per three staff members setting. Practitioners of EAAT need to remember that in the ABA setting the instructor (not the child) is the leader. A very important part of ABA is a reward for the correct response. The reward can have different forms. It can be a token, or a favorite exercise, a sensory stimulation that the child likes, or the ability to choose the next game. The team needs to remember that unless a behavior creates danger to the participant, horse or, staff negative behaviors or incorrect responses should be ignored. Negative attention is also a kind of attention and it may actually reinforce a reaction. Simply repeating the exercise and not concentrating on the negative is the way to go. It is also important that in order to succeed in life generalization of acquired skills must exist. Taking the skills learned in the EAAT setting and transitioning them to real life situations can be very beneficial.

Resources:

http://www.apbahome.net/

http://www.autismspeaks.org/what-autism/treatment/applied-behavior-analysis-aba

www.abainternational.org [The Association for Behavior Analysis International]

www.apa.org/crsppp/archivbehav.html [American Psychological Association Archival Description of Behavioral Psychology]

www.apbahome.net [The Association of Professional Behavior Analysts]

www.bacb.com

www.BACB.com [Behavior Analyst Certification Board]

www.behavior.org

www.behavior.org [Cambridge Center for Behavioral Studies]

CHAPTER SEVEN

Developmental Individual Difference Relation-Based Intervention (DIR- "Floortime")

DIR was developed by Stanley Greenspan and Serena Wieder. It approaches treatment from a developmental point of view. The basic concept of this model can be summarized in that an adult can help a child expand his circles of communication by meeting him at his developmental level and building on his strengths. The therapy very often takes place in the form of play on the floor (so it is also known as Floortime approach). It is important to notice that Floortime is play with a purpose and it is one of many ways that a DIR can be utilized. It is not an interchangeable name for DIR.

DIR is about focusing on strengthening and then building upon the emotional bond of the child with his or her caregiver. The emphasis is put on the individuality of each child and adult relationship. This approach works with the whole family and not just with the child.

DIR utilizes existing therapies and develops new approaches to encourage children to pass through six hierarchal functional-developmental milestones:

1. *Self regulation and interest in the world.* This first stage brings the ability to stay calm and regulated and to share attention. Usually children achieve this stage in the first three months of life. The ability to use all the senses to gather information from the environment and self-regulation enable successful interaction with the environment. Without them the child cannot progress to higher developmental levels.

2. *Intimacy.* The second milestone which naturally occurs between two and nine moths focuses on engagement and relatedness. Engagement in the DIR terminology means to be related to another, not engaged in some self-absorbed interest. At this stage we want the child to

focus on us. The relation that is created can be used to build onto the child's next developmental stages.

3. *Two-way communication.* The beginning of communication is displayed by gestures that can be used both to initiate communication and to respond to communication from others. Usually occurring between four to nine months, this is the beginning of real conversation. The child starts to understand the meaning of the interaction with others. Not mastering this milestone leads to problems with reading nonverbal cues. Children may require outside help with initiating and sustaining meaningful interaction.

4. *Complex communication.* The next step in development of communication skills, problem solving, co-regulation, and interactions usually occurs between nine to eighteen months of life. The child starts to communicate wishes and intentions by putting together gestures. He or she can also better understand gestures of other people. The child starts appreciating the power of communication. The communication feels like a flow. This fluidity and close connection are essential for moving to the next level.

5. *Emotional ideas.* This stage normally occurs between eighteenth to thirtieth month and manifests itself through, among others things, representational play. This is the phase in which abstract thinking begins to take place. The child starts utilizing ideas and words in creative and meaningful ways. At this level the child starts to enter the phase in which he or she can stop relying only on memory to navigate the world around them. Symbols are starting to form in his or her mind.

6. *Emotional thinking.* This is the stage in which building of logical bridges between ideas occurs. It occurs between thirty to forty-eight months of live. The child develops a greater understanding of self and others and of how the

actions of one person can affect another. He or she can take ideas presented by someone, think about them, add it to their own thoughts and put out a response that is a mix of ideas of both parties. Verbal and special skills increase and higher level of emotions start to form.

Incorporating DIR into EAATs and vice versa

In EAAT setting it is important to find out which stage of development the child is currently at. Depending on the level, the structure of the session will be different. The child who is in the first stage will probably need a lot of sensory integration exercises and one-on-one contact. If that is the case, a hippotherapy setting would be the most appropriate for the client at this level. The second stage of development will bring a slow introduction of new people, new horses, and maybe a beginning of a group class or a presence of a different rider in the arena. At this level a slow transition to THR riding may take place. The third stage could include working on involvement in the lesson. We may start allowing the child to make decisions (give choices) and to communicate its needs and wants. Communication can be both verbal and non verbal. The fourth stage may include continuation of work on sensory integration and communication. This is the time where we may start to allow the child to make choices and to communicate choices. Introduction of group activities and team skills may take place at this level. At the fifth stage we would include work on representational ideas and play. The therapist or instructor can start to engage the child by asking him or her to describe world and feelings during and after session. Activities may include talking about particular objects or the horse. If the client is in the last stage of development we may continue to work on understanding emotions and connecting emotions. Games may include distinguishing between I/mine and his/yours. Talking about the horse, what they like, what would they feel if something happened should also support the development at this stage.

Resources

www.ICDL.com

Home.sprintmail.com/-
hanettevance/floor_time.htm#ToSixDevelopmentalMilstones

CHAPTER EIGHT

Miller Method

A method created by Arnold Miller for children with ASD and with severe learning disorders, the Miller Method addresses children's body organization, social interaction, communication and representation issues in both clinical and classroom settings[32]. It tries to close gaps in how a child perceives and thinks about the world and in the child's developmental progress by using the *system concept.* This concept utilizes a desire to complete units of behavior to teach new things. "*A System* is a coherent organization (functional or nonfunctional) of behavior involving an object, event or person"[33]. It can be small and simple or big and complex. In essence, systems are organized "chunks" of behavior. At the beginning of development, the child doesn't have control over the systems. It closely reacts to the environment. As the development progresses and children become more and more aware of the distinction between themselves and their immediate surroundings they gain control over the systems. In time the systems can be combined in new ways that permit problem solving, social exchanges, and communication with themselves and others.

Children with developmental delays can get stuck in the early developmental stage or progress at an uneven rate. The concept of systems plays a role in restoring normal development using the Miller Method in two ways. First of all using the repetitive behaviors (systems) that the child already has, it introduces new behaviors and activities and transforms the system into functional behaviors. Second, it teaches the children new behaviors which they have not been able to develop by themselves. The Miller Method utilizes the power of an *interrupted system* to teach functional communication and general expansion of a child's awareness of the world around him.

---

[32] http://autism.millermethod.org/

[33] "Shore, S.M., Rastelli, L.G. (2006 p 161

According to Miller's theory, during a typical development the child passes through five stages. In the first four stages the child is reacting to the environment or events. In the final stage the child has an element of control. The five stages of typical development are:

1. *Orienting* – In this stage the child makes initial contact with a stimulus within the surroundings. A child looking at a toy or noticing the presence of a horse, instructor, etc. would be an example or behavior at this stage.

2. *Engagement of stimulus* comes next. The child begins to interact with the object or a person (ex. petting a horse, brushing the horse, reaching for a toy, touching a toy).

3. *Formation of system* occurs when the child begins to act on the stimulus or develops another repetitive, predictable, organized unit of behavior around it. The child has the system fully integrated if the behavior continues on its own or the child makes an attempt to continue the behavior after the system is interrupted.

4. *Formation of ritual* when silent sensory input from an aspect of the system activates the entire behavior. A child who can form a system is dominated by the system; it lacks the ability to choose whether to engage in the system. So if we present a child with a ring it will attempt to put it on a horse's ear, even though it may have a choice of putting it on a hand.

5. *Repertoire* – the final stage at which the child has the element of choice. Presented with a selection of toys or options it will be able to pick a different toy. This gradually developing function is based on the switch from external events to internal ones. The child learns to make choices.

Millers Method utilizes elevation structures[34]. They are to help raise the child's awareness of the world around them. Children can focus

---

[34] The example of such structure can be found at
http://www.cognitivedesigns.com/playthings.html

better when placed on elevated objects. Such positioning limits "spin-off" into space and raises the child to face the adult at the same level.

Miller's Method in EAAT's

Utilizing Miller's Method in EAAT's can be a very natural approach. First we introduce the child to the horse and to the surrounding. This would be an equivalent of the orienting phase. The child naturally progresses to petting the horse and interacting with objects in its proximity. For example, the client is playing with brushes and toys but not necessarily using them to perform given tasks; just exploring. Thus a simple system forms. Presented with a task the child knows how to complete it. For example when given a ring he or she knows to put it on the horse's ear. The system can also be much simpler and just consist of getting on the horse when seeing one or using a brush to brush the horse. At this level the child will insist on continuing within the system and may not be happy if any changes are introduced. This can be seen, for example, if a client refuses to ride a different horse or doesn't like a change in routine. Next a ritual or a routine is crated in the form of a whole session. The child knows that after coming to the barn he or she will put a helmet on, help brushing the horse, mount, do warm ups, do a series of exercises or games, dismounts and says goodbye to the horse and staff. On a much simpler level he or she may run to the ramp without seeing the horse just because they are in the barn. The last and final stage takes place when the child is able to make choices. Presented with a choice of mounting from a ramp or a mounting block it may pick the unfamiliar one. Another example is a choice of an old or new game or activity, or a choice of gait.

It is worth mentioning that a ramp and a horse by their nature form an elevated structure and promote awareness of the world around the child. It is also worth highlighting that the Miller Method is very effective with children who are nonverbal and on the more severe end of the spectrum.

Resources:

http://www.millermethod.org/

Miller A, Chretien K. (2007) *The Miller Method. Developing the Capacities of Children on the Autism Spectrum.* Philadelphia: Jessica Kingsley Publishers

Miller A, Eller-Miller E. (1989). *From Ritual to Repertoire. A Cognitive-Developmental Systems Approach with Behavior-Disordered Children.* NY: John Wiley & Sons.

Shore, S.M., Rastelli, L.G. ((2006). Understanding Autism for Dummies. Hoboken, NJ: Wiley Publishing, Inc.

CHAPTER NINE

RDI- Relationship Development Intervention

Developed by Steven Gutstein and Rachel Sheely, RDI is a parent-based approach which concentrates on difficulties in cognition, emotion, communication and social interaction. It is a family based intervention that tries to enabling people with autism to have a higher quality of life. The RDI process encourages the child to participate in experience sharing interactions. Instrumental social interactions that are scripted and have a specific end point treat people as "instruments" or means to the end. The challenge is to lead the child toward experience-sharing interactions where common experience is created. It introduces novelty, joy and curiosity into the child's life. According to this method the best way to achieve the goal is to develop dynamic intelligence. There are two types of intelligence: dynamic and static. Static intelligence is anything that has a clear right or wrong answer. The outcome is always the same, nothing changes. Static skills include labeling, academics, requesting, social scripts, following directions and memorization. Most people living with ASD function pretty well in these type of situations. Dynamic intelligence is an ability to manage situation that have an element of uncertainty. Most people who are not on the spectrum seem to possess the ability to solve problems, share experiences with others, develop curiosity, empathy and look at problems from another person's point of view. In all these situation there is no right or wrong answer, and no way to predict a very specific outcome. This type of intelligence is very rare in individuals with ASD.

RDI tries to develop six areas of emotional intelligence which in turn will allow them to join in on the pleasures of life[35]. These areas are:

- ***Emotional referencing*** which through different means of communication gives a person the ability to understand how the other person is feeling.

---

[35] Information found on RDI Web site (www.ridconnect.com)

- *Social coordination* which is the ability to feel the same emotions as another person and ability to straighten out a misunderstanding or prevent lack of communication.
- *Declarative language* which is an ability to make statements about our world and surroundings through different means of communication. It is our basic way of connecting with the world.
- *Flexible thinking* in the ability of flexible cognitive shifting – going with the flow of events even when they are unpredictable would be one example of flexible thinking.
- *Relational information processing* is the ability to co-regulate one's behavior and reaction depending on the surrounding situation.

Based on those six areas of competence the creators of RDI formed eight guiding principles for enabling children with autism to more successfully interact with the world.

1. **Building a strong foundation** – the RDI program is broken down into systematic and measurable objectives. Because it is a parent-based intervention, parents work out their own objectives prior to the assignment of any objectives for the child. The parent's readiness to begin the work of reestablishing the guided participation relationship is a key element in this approach. Next, the goals for child with ASD and for the siblings are established.
2. **Developing a user-friendly environment** - each child's capabilities are evaluated and modifications to the environment and pace of the program are set in such a way as to provide a safe environment in which the child can explore new ways of interacting.
3. **Implementing guided participation through a "master" and "apprentice" relationship** - working with a parent or another person who is significant in the child's life, the child explores and develops new ways of understanding his or her environment. During this process the child moves from following the master to more and more inde-

pendent dealings with new and confusing situations. The final goal is for the child to become independent to the point where he or she can deal with their "master" on equal terms.

4. **Improving personal episodic memory** - Episodic memory allows us to remember a given event through its emotional aspects. The memory is associated with an emotion and then regularly reviewed through telling stories or daily reflections.

5. **Building motivation for dynamic systems** – the desire to experience emotions stored throughout episodic memory can serve as a motivator to repeat the activities.

6. **Changing communication** - RDI encourages the use of declarative rather than imperative statements. The declarative statements focus on emotional states rather than questions or demands to modify a given behavior. They are used to predict, reflect and regulate interaction and to demonstrate curiosity. Examples of declarative statements can be "We can do it" "Oh that's so exciting!" and very often used imperative statements are "Look at me!" "Don't do that!" "Say thank you!"

7. **Creating opportunities for practice** – making teachable moments out of ordinary and unplanned events is called incidental learning. In RDI this concept is so important that it is taken so far as to assist parents in adapting their schedule to increase the number of incidental learning events.

8. **Progressive generalization** - as children achieve proficiency and success in earlier systems and goals the foundation for participating in more complex activities is created. One can introduce different settings, situations, and people. The distractions that were purposefully removed from the environment beforehand can now be reintroduced so that the child can develop the skills necessary for focusing on what's important.

RDI in an EAAT's setting

Introducing the RDI model of support into EAAT is not difficult. Team collaboration, working with parents, and making sure that the program is aligned with the goals of the child should be part of any program. Following the eight guiding principle will allow any EAAT program to be more successful.

As mentioned before, breaking down each goal and setting measurable objectives is good practice for any program. Good lesson plans and an appropriate therapy plan will form a strong foundation for growth and development. The modification of the environment and making sure that it safe for the client and horse is also considered a basic step in any program creation. Making the environment and lessons interesting and motivating for the client allows growth and assures a higher level of participation.

Implementing guided participation through a "master" and apprentice relationship in the EAAT setting can have many forms. The basic instruction of how to tack up a horse or a group lesson can have a format of a "master" –"apprentice" relationship. Another possibility for implementation of this concept is the creation of a volunteer program that will enable a person with ASD to work alongside with a "neurotypical" peer or adult supervisor. In all of my previous positions I established a "Special Volunteer" program where people with special needs volunteer at the barn supervised by the support staff who work with them every day. It is a win-win situation. The volunteers are able to learn new skills that can later be transferred to everyday life or used on resumes, the community gets to experience integration, and the center has more helpful hands.

Interacting with horses is a very emotional experience for most clients. It is a natural way of improving personal episodic memory and an easy way to build motivation. Our clients don't see the sessions as therapy sessions. They perceive most activities as "time with a horse" or "time at the barn". The motivation to repeat the experience is in most cases tremendous.

Good communication skills are necessary for any person who works in any therapeutic setting. Building on positives and emphasizing strong sides of our clients as well as good communication with the parents and care givers should be a common practice for all EAAT instructors. The therapist and instructors should remember that we are all playing on the same team and have a common goal. There is no "us" and "them". Forming a team and being a part of a team working for the client will also lead to creating more opportunities for practice and generalization of skills across different settings. If the EAAT program is alienated from IEP the client has more chances to work on the same concepts across all of the activities during the day. The barn can also create great opportunity for growth and participation in activities with "neuro-typical" peers and colleges. Progressing from hippotherapy, through therapeutic riding, to Special Olympics, Para - Olympics or main-stream competitions allows for fluid transition and more opportunity for practice and progress.

Resources

http://www.rdiconnect.com/

Gutstein S. (2009). *The RDI Book:Forging New Pathways for Autsim, Asperger's and PDD with the Relationship Development Intervention Program.* Houston: Connection Center Publishing.

CHAPTER TEN

TEACCH
Treatment and Education of Autistic and Communication Handicapped Children (TEACCH)

TEACCH is more of a philosophy than a concrete treatment approach. It draws on different therapeutic approaches in various combinations, depending on the children needs. TEACCH was created in North Carolina at Chapel Hill in early 1970. It emphasizes understanding the characteristics of people with autism as a basis for arranging their environments to maximize success. TEACCH concentrates on the strong and positive aspects of a given child and not on the problematic areas. The program is built individually for each child and is based on existing skills and interests.

The practitioners of TEACCH always try to work with - not against - autism. Their structured teaching approach is based on understanding how people with autism think and function. According to The TEACCH Approach to Autism Spectrum Disorders (2004), by Gary B. Mesibove, Victoria Shea, and Eric Shopler (Springer) all individual programs should include the following elements:

> ➤ **Organization of physical environment** - Clear physical boundaries help the child with understanding where they need to be and what they need to do. Visual cues are placed in each room to remind the child what the purpose of each area is.

> ➤ **Predictable sequence of events** - Recurring sequences of events lessen anxiety levels. Students should have a schedule both during school/therapy sessions and during leisure time. This corresponds to calendars and "to-do-lists" that are used by many people.

> ➤ **Routines with flexibility** – People with autism often crave routines. Providing them with healthy routines helps prevent

developing dysfunctional routines. Practitioners can also implement slight changes to build flexibility into the routine. This prepares the person for functioning in the world that is constantly changing and can be unpredictable to some degree.

➢ **Visual schedules** – Since most people with autism tend to process visual information better, providing a picture or written schedule increases the chances of a person doing what was planed and communicated earlier. It can also lessen anxiety during transition periods. Visual schedules also provide the feeling of security and competence without constant supervision of an adult.

➢ **Visually structured activities** - It is easier to engage a person with autism by providing them with something that is touchable or visible. According to TEACCH practitioners, during each task a person with autism should be provided with:

  ▪ *Instruction* - example of finished work, visualization of each step if needed. A photo of a prepared sandwich followed by a series of photos showing how to make a sandwich, for example.

  ▪ *Organization* – Orderly space, easy access to materials, and providing only the materials that are needed for given tasks makes the life of a person with autism much easier.

  ▪ *Clarity* – materials should be categorized and color coded.

➢ **Work/activity systems** - Provide an easier way to approach a given task. It is a systematic approach to organize all tasks. Each description should have following elements:

• *What?* – what is the task, what are its parts?

• *How much?* – How many times does the given task needs to be done, how many repetitions?

- *What progress have I made and when am I finished?* – A way to measure progress either by time or by number of finished tasks.

- *What happens next?* - What will happen after completion of a task? Transition to a different room or a different station, for example.

The TEACCH Approach is a very practical way of helping people with autism become more successful in interactions with their environment and other people. It can also be utilized during EAAT's.

Incorporating TEACCH into EAAT's practice

The systematic and structured way of dealing with each situation that is utilized in TEACCH can be very easily incorporated during any form of activities involving horses. All horses and most human being like to have some level of routines to follow. Structuring each session and organizing the physical environment in a way which will benefit both the client and the horse should not be difficult. Organization of physical environment, for example should already be taking place in any barn providing EAAT's. The environment around horses needs to be neat, clean and, safe. This means all unnecessary equipment and machinery need to be stored away and out of reach. This is an equivalent of clarity and organization. The door of the ring needs to be closed at all times if there is a participant on a horse according to the standards of PATH International. This provides a distinctive space to work and a separate space to mount a horse. Most EAAT sessions follow a routine and have a somewhat predictable sequence of events. As for visual cues, using a board with a schedule or having pictures of activities are common practice during hippotherapy and therapeutic riding sessions. If the client does not have his or her own portable board one can be easily made with a piece of cardboard and Velcro's.

Resources:

www.teacch.com

CHAPTER ELEVEN

SCERTS
Social Communication Emotional Regulation Transactional Support Model (SCERTS)

SCERTS is another example of a research based educational model for working with children and their families. It utilizes existing approaches to best match the child's needs. Like TEACCH, it is more of a philosophy than a specific kind of intervention. SCERTS practitioners concentrate on social communication, preventing problem behaviors, and developing relationships. The families, educators, and therapists work as a team. SCERTS is also a life-long model that can be used from initial diagnosis, throughout the school years and beyond. It is also very flexible and adaptable for various settings, which makes it easy to adapt for EAAT.

The SCERTS model has three components[36]:

"SC"- social communication - focuses on development of spontaneous, functional communication, expressing emotions, and relationships with other people. According to the SCERTS philosophy social communication competence has a direct influence on relationships and living within a given community. The emphasis is placed on child-initiated communication in an everyday setting and in semi-structured activities. The practitioners encourage requesting, protesting, sharing attention, sharing emotion, and sharing experiences. Later on the emphasis also progresses to the importance of considering someone else's perspective, taking turns, and solving problems with communication. The two major areas of communication in the SCERTS program are:

---

[36] Prizant B., Wetherby A., Rubin E., Laurent A. (2010)

> *Join attention*[37], which is the idea of sharing a reference point with another person. Knowing what the other person is pointing at is an example of joint attention.

> *Symbol use*, which refers to how a person communicates. There are three levels of symbols that can be used to communicate. Pre-symbolic stage refers to using gestures or objects to communicate. The symbolic stage which utilizes signs, pictures, and symbols is next. The third stage is functional verbal communication. Ideally, the child should be able to switch between all three modalities as needed in a given situation. For example, pointing and using other gestures in a very loud room would be more appropriate than speaking to the other person. Establishing good communication allows the person with ASD to have their needs successfully met and to reduce the reliance on unacceptable or challenging behaviors as a model of communication.

The second component of the SCERTS Model and the "ER" part of acronym in the "SCERTS" is Emotional Regulation.

According to the SCERTS practitioners, Emotional Regulation stands for "the development of the ability to maintain a well-regulated emotional stage to cope with everyday stress, and to be most available for learning and interacting."[38] It is basically the ability to ignore outside distractions and outside input from the environment. Unfortunately people on the ASD spectrum very often have difficulties with regulating their internal emotional state or ignoring the outside environment. SCERTS teaches people on the ASD spectrum how to seek out and respond to support in the three areas of regulation:

1. **Mutual regulation** - occurs when the person with ASD, when faced with overwhelming amount of stress, requests or accepts assistance from another person to help regain composure. For example when the person is overly stimulated in a noisy room he or she may ask to leave the room for a quieter environment. A good EAAT example would be to ask the side

---

[37] Shore, S.M., Rastelli, L.G. (2006)
[38] Prizant B., Wetherby A., Rubin E., Laurent A. (2010). p. 315

walker to remove a hand from the leg if the touch was getting too overwhelming.

2. **Self-regulation** - "refers to educating the person how to remain at an optimal level of arousal when confronted with a potentially stressful situation."[39] An example of self-regulation can be carrying a set of ear plugs in case the room might become too loud or wearing gloves in order to reduce sensitivity to the touch when holding rains.

3. **Recovery from extreme dysregulation** – refers to the process of actions that need to be undertaken after a person becomes so over-stimulated that he or she either has a breakdown or shuts down. Ideally the person will be taught how to avoid and prevent dysregulation, but every person should know how to recover from one in case it occurs. Seeking a quiet place or carrying notes that can be passed to officials are examples of dealing with extreme dysregulation.

The third part of the SCERTS – the "TS" – stands for Transactional Support. This is the part that connects the first two elements of the system by teaching other people (parents, teachers, therapists, members of the community) how to help and advocate for people living with ASD. As a community we can provide support in four areas: interpersonal, in formal and informal settings in all areas of life, by helping families by providing opportunities to incorporate the system into their family, in education and community systems and by supporting professionals and other service providers.

Utilizing SCERTS within EAAT

As a model that utilizes already existing techniques SCERTS is very easily implemented within the various EAAT modalities. First, it is based on a proper evaluation of the client's needs and an assessment of his or her situation. The client is also an active participant in setting up his or her own program. In EAAT enjoying the activities and willingness to participate in the exercises are

---

[39] Shore, S.M., Rastelli, L.G. (2006) p 175

prerequisites to effective participation. The aspect that I would like to emphasize most in utilizing the SCERTS model is the importance of working as a team and establishing a support network. The team work is important on two levels. First of all, each center should have a team of professionals that can assist the riding instructors and therapists in establishing the plan of action. In a perfect world the team would consist of an occupational therapist, physical therapist, psychologist, and a speech therapist. This doesn't mean that each client should be working with all these therapists at once during riding sessions. Optimally all of these specialists should have an input during the planning phase and should be available for consultations if the need arises. The second part of the team aspect is the team that is already in place and working for and with a given client. The riding instructor or hippotherapist should become an integral part of this team and should have access to all the information that may help with designing a safe and effective plan for the client.

It is also important to point out that all three main components of SCERTS are worth implementing in programs of all EAAT participants. Social communication, emotional regulation and transactional support are necessary components of social life for all people, not only those that are on the ASD spectrum.

Resources:

http://www.barryprizant.com/

Prizant B., Wetherby A., Rubin E., Laurent A. (2010). The SCERTS Model. In ed: Ken Siri, Tony Lyons *Cutting Therapies for Autism 2011-2011*. Skyhorse Publishing

Shore, S.M., Rastelli, L.G. ((2006). *Understanding Autism for Dummies*. Hoboken, NJ: Wiley Publishing, Inc.

www.scerts.com

CHAPTER TWELVE

The Son-Rise Program

The Son Rise Program was created by Barry Nail Kaufman and Sa-
mahria Lyte Kaufman when their son, Raun was diagnosed as severe-
ly and incurably autistic. They were first to suggest that children with
autism diagnoses had the potential for extraordinary healing and
growth.

The program is based on the assumption that "The child/person
shows us the way to his/her world and then we can show him/her the
way to the outside world[40]". The philosophy of the program is based
on the fact that the bond between people is the basis for growth and
education. It also assumes that autism is a relational, interactional
disorder. At its core, autism is a neurological challenge which causes
children to have difficulty relating and connecting to those around
them. Most of their so-called behavioral challenges stem from this relational deficit. The main goal is to create interpersonal bonds and
social interactions. The first and most important element that is taught
during the training is joining. Joining means that one joins, rather than
stops, a child's repetitive, exclusive and ritualistic behaviors. When the
child accepts you into their world and you are showing interest in what
the child is doing you can create the strong bond around the common
interest. In return the child starts to show real interest in your person.
The interest of the child creates the door to support growth and education. The self-motivation of each child is used to generate interest in
an activity. Each subject/activity is presented in such a way as to be
most attractive for the child. The activities are built around interest and
skills that the child already has (ex. trains). It provides higher motivation and a will to cooperate. At the same time the material is integrated, not just learned, which in turn leads to generalizations and
spontaneous use of learned skills.

The social goals of the Son-Rise Program (communication, eye contact, interactive attention spans, and flexibility) are taught through Developmental Mode. These goals are always addressed before

---

[40] Raun Kaufman (2010) p. 344.

academic goals. The program assumes that the academic knowledge is important but it will not help the person overcome the main problem which is difficulties creating a social bond with other people. These social bonds are more important than knowledge. The goal is to overcome the social difficulties, not compensate for them.

Another very important part of the Son-Rise Program, one that is definitely worth mentioning and applying within other modalities, is the attitude towards the child. Parents and the therapist should have a non-judgmental, inviting, and optimistic attitude toward the child. This attitude will help the child to feel safe and relax, which in turn will help him or her to build relationship and share feelings and be relaxed enough to learn. Parents participating in the Son-Rise program spend time working with their emotional and attitudinal challenges. I would like to emphasize that no matter what therapeutic modality the family decides to undertake the "help yourself before helping others" and "take care of yourself so you can help others" attitude is very important. The life of any parents is difficult, but a life of a family with a special child can be even more stressful[41].

Son-Rise Program and EAAT

Applying the Son-Rise program in a barn setting may present a challenge. The most basic principal of this modality, which is following the child and not enforcing any rules, may be difficult to implement in a situation where rules are necessary for safety reasons. It doesn't mean that it is impossible, however. If the child is happy around horses and has no problem with putting on a helmet, mounted activities can be slowly introduced. If a child is able to communicate or join with a therapist and accept different activities on a horse, we may set up a set of activities around the arena and allow the child to choose which one he or she wants to do next. If the child is severally autistic but accepts being on a horse, the therapist can go on a trail ride and join in whatever activity the child does on a horse (ex: touching the horse, rocking while moving, just being next to the child and horse). There is

---

[41] In my personal practice I provide life coaching and support for parents of children on ASD spectrum. For more information about this program go to www.helptogrowinstitute.com

a big chance that the child will first start noticing the horse and connecting with the horse and only later on may shift his or her attention to the therapist. This is called passive riding and its effects are described in the next chapter, which focuses on research in the field of EAAT and autism and on practical solutions to some of the challenges that can be worked on during EAAT's.

Resources

Raun Kaufman (2010). Son-Rise Program In ed.: Ken Siri, Tony Lyons *Cutting Therapies for Autism 2011-2011*. Skyhorse Publishing

www.autismtreatment.org

PART FOUR

HORSE AS A THERAPIST OF AUTISTIC CHILD

CHAPTER THIRTEEN

Does it work? Research in autism and EAAT

So far we have discussed the theoretical basis of EAAT in industry and research patterning for different disabilities. But how do we know that this approach works for the people with ASD? There is not much research about EAAT and autism, but some exist. Below are two example of scientific proof that horse therapy is a great modality to support innervations for people on the autism spectrum.

SYNCHRONIZATION OF SENSORY MOTOR REACTIONS IN CHILDREN WITH AUTISM DURING HIPPOTHERAPY

As part of my PhD study at the Pilsudsky's University of Physical Education in Warsaw, Poland (2002-2007) I conducted research on short and mid- term influence of hippotherapy on children with autism.

This research had 3 objectives

1.   To evaluate the influence of hippotherapy on:

- Motor skills of children with autism.
- Sensory motor synchronization in children with autism.

2.   To describe the influence of the horse's walk on an autistic child that is seating passively.

3.   To evaluate the influence of hippotherapy on the level of social development and self –care skills of children with autism.

The research questions where as follow

1)   Did the hippotherapy program have an influence on the exercised motor skills of autistic children?

2)   Did the hippotherapy program have an influence on sensory motor synchronization (particularly eye hand coordination) of autistic children?

3)   Did the hippotherapy program have an influence on the development of social and self-care skills of autistic children?

4)   How did the horse's walk on a straight line influence the change in the autistic child's:

- Position of the head;
- Center of gravity;
- The size of the angle between:

      - a the lower leg and thigh

      - b the thigh and the trunk

      - d the trunk and the head

Methodology:

There were two parts to the research that had separate research groups and methodology.

  1. Research Groups:

A. Part one consisted of 6 single case studies of boys who participated in 18 sessions of hippotherapy. One of the boys stopped the participation do to unrelated health problems after 12 sessions, and 2 resigned after 4 sessions. The final analyses included the data collected from 3 boys. All of them understood verbal comments at the age from 7 to 9 years old. Autism was also the only diagnosis that these boys had.

Patient 1- C.S. d.b. 08.1997, poor speech.

Patient 2- P.K. d.b. 07.1996, very good speech.

Patient 3- K.Z d.b. 08.1998, very good speech

B. Patients participating in motion analysis:

In the second part of the research, out of 18 boys who participated in summer camp and whose parents allowed us to record part of the hippotherapy sessions, 6 were able to sit on the horse motionless long enough to obtain material that allowed motion analyses. These were boys in age ranging from 5-7 years old with different levels of autistic tendencies. All of them were able to react to verbal commands and did not have any other diagnosis.

2.   Research methodology:

The research was conducted in a following way:

A. Case study:

-First examination: Vineland Scale, interview with parents.

-18 hippotherapy sessions 0.5 hours during two school semesters. Video-recording of some sessions (1, 5,10,15,18).

-Second examination: Vineland Scale, interview with parents, analysis of video recordings.

The research utilized Vineland Adaptive Behavior Scale (VABS, Sparrow et all., 1984). It was first created in 1965 and modified and extended in 1984 by team of Sary Sparrow. There is no Polish Standardization of this scale.

Currently the VABS have three versions:

1. Interview- questionnaire, which has 297 questions

2. Extended interview, which has 577 questions

3. 244 task (80% are the same as in the interview version)

In this research the Interview –questionnaire version was used.

The scale has four subscales:

- Communication
- Independence in everyday life
- Motor skills
- Socialization

The scale can be used by a psychologist, social worker or trained personnel. The interview is conducted with an adult who is very familiar with the child and his/her behaviors. The interview takes from 20 to 60 minutes to complete. The answers cannot be read to the responder. The goal is to catch what the child can usually accomplish. The results are assigned the following points:

-2 points if the activity is performed in the normal and satisfactory manner (even if the child has an opportunity to engage in the activity only sporadically);

-1 point if the activity is only partially performed or sometimes performed. This gate is allowed only for the marked questions;

-0 points, if the activity is never accomplished, because the child cannot perform given activity or someone else is executing it for the child.

-N (not applicable) –the activity could not be performed do to the external conditions.

-DK (don't know)- the respondent doesn't know or is not able to answer.

To establish developmental age of the child the questions are continued to the point in which none or three consecutive activities that the child was involved in were not completed.

iii) Video recording of motor activity during hippotherapy sessions

a)   Video recording of the hippotherapy sessions

Out of 18 sessions that each of 5 clients attended 5 were recorded (1st, 5th, 10th, 15th, and 18th). Reaction times and behaviors were observed and coded. The video was captured with the use of digital camera Sony DCR –TRV 19E. The following measures were coded:

- eye contact;
- undesirable behaviors;
- keeping balance;
- grasping with hands;
- throwing to a target;

- putting on and taking of rings;
- exercise "lying back";
- exercise change of position "Mill";
- exercise "lying on the neck";
- exercise "Over the barrel".

b) Motion analysis of the body posture of patients sitting on a horse which is traveling on a straight line at walk

During a passive hippotherapy session a reference quadrant was marked on the wall (1m by 1 m). This reference quadrant allowed us to establish a reference scale of the picture on the computer screen in relation to real life dimensions. Perpendicular to the wall at the distance of 5 m a Sony DCR-TRV 19 E camera was placed on a tripod. The clients were videotaped from the left side while passively sitting on the horse that was walking in a straight line.

-system APAS (Ariel Performance Analysis System) by ARIEL (USA);

Methods of evaluation:

a)   Analysis of behaviors and tasks that the children engaged in during therapeutic sessions on the horse

After completion of the whole therapeutic cycle each aspect of child's behavior was analyzed and the pre and post test results of Vineland Scale were compared. Also each video recorded session was analyzed including reaction time and behavioral changes.

b)   Motion analysis of the autistic child's posture during walk on a horse on a straight line:

For this part of research the APAS (Ariel performance Analysis System) was utilized. It is a video based motion analysis system which provides objective biomechanical data. Video registration for this kind of analysis must meet two requirements:

- Each frame must be a separate take no matter what the speed of registration is;

- The proportions of the registered film to the real life scale must be known.

To make the calculation possible the human is deciphered as a simple animation or stick diagram. The final results showed the change of values of angles (in frontal plane and function of consecutive film frames) of:

- α – lower leg and the thigh
- β – the thigh and the trunk
- δ – the trunk and the head
- and the position of the head and center of gravity as a function of consecutive film frames.

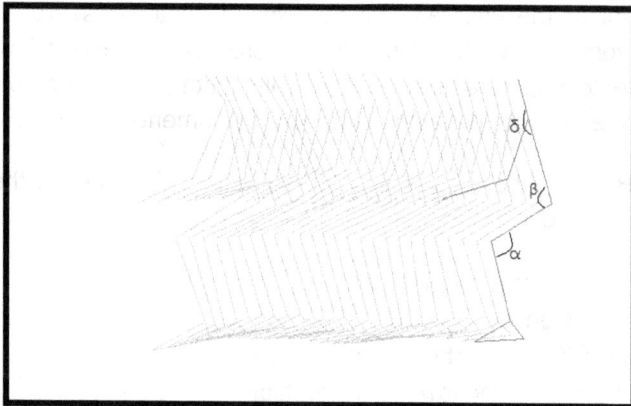

Pic.3 The geometrical model of a child sitting on a horse and the considered angles.

The research answered the following questions:

1) Did the use of the hippotherapy program have an influence on the exercised motor skills of autistic children?

The therapeutic program, to some degree, had a positive influence on some of the motor skills of autistic patients. The progress and the types of exercise used were different for each patient.

2)   Did the use of a hippotherapy program have an influence on sensory motor synchronization (particularly hand-eye coordination) of autistic children?

In some cases, the therapeutic program had a positive influence on synchronization of sensory motor reactions (particularly hand-eye co-ordination). The degree of progress was dependent on the initial state of the participant.

3) Did the use of hippotherapy program have an influence on development of social and self-care skills of autistic children?

If one uses the right exercises, the frequency and duration of undesirable behaviors could be decreased.

4) All of the children that participated in the research showed improvement in skills, including self-care skills. However, it was not possible to separate the influence of hippotherapy from other factors, such as natural development and environmental factors.

5) How did the horse's walk in a straight line influence the change in the autistic child's:

- Position of the head;
- Center of gravity;
- The size of the angle between:
    - a the lower leg and thigh
    - b the thigh and the trunk
    - d the trunk and the head

An autistic child, passively sitting on a walking horse, has passive, uncontrolled movements, and because of that such children should have an individual exercise program while riding.

5)   During passive therapy on a walking horse the head had moved in the frontal plane. This may suggest the presence of a stimulation of vagues nerve and self-regulation of vagal and vestibular systems.

THERAPEUTIC HORSEBACK RIDING IN CHILDREN WITH AUTISM SPECTRUM DISORDER

Another current research project focused exclusively on TR and autism was presented by Amy Shoffner and Robin Gabriels in STRIDES MAGAZINE in 2011. The project was a collaboration between the Colorado Therapeutic Riding Center in Longmont and Children's Hospital in Denver.

In the study 41 children age 6-16 participated in 10 consecutive weekly TR group lessons. All participants had IQ above 40. Each group consisted of 3 to 4 children and the lessons were taught by an Advance PATH International Certified Instructor. Pre and post testing included:

> ➤ Diagnostic and IQ screening evaluations
> ➤ Screening at Colorado Therapeutic Riding Center (CTRC) to:
>   ▪ Assess horsemanship skills and level of functioning
>   ▪ Assign to appropriate THR group based on level of functioning
> ➤ Exclusion based on an inability to interact with the horse
> ➤ Evaluation by OT and research assistants.
> ➤ Pre- and post-THR evaluation within one month prior to and following participation in ten weeks of THR lessons to assess motor and adaptive skills

Methodological tools included:

- Aberrant Behavior Checklist-Community (ABC-C)
- Vineland Adaptive Behavior Scales-II (VABS-II)
- Bruininks-Oseretsky Test of Motor Proficiency (BOT-II)
- Sensory Integration and Praxis Test (SIPT)

The intervention included:

- THR weekly interventions
- Intervention followed skill progression and objectives
- Horse and side-walker volunteers were consistent for each participant

- Picture schedule of lesson activities were presented before each lesson to parents and children.

The caregivers completed ABC-C pre- and post- 10-weeks of THR.

Sixteen children participated in 10 week waitlist control group before entering THR study and were evaluated at the beginning and the end of the 10 weeks. In comparison to control group the therapeutic group showed:

- ✓ Significant improvements in ABC-C subscale scores for irritability, hyperactivity, lethargy, Stereotype, inappropriate speech ($p < 0.01$)
- ✓ Mixed effects ANOVA found ABC-C improvements significant after three weeks for Irritability, Hyperactivity, Lethargy and Stereotype
- ✓ Significant improvement ($p<0.01$) in BOT-II and SIPT Verbal Praxis
- ✓ Significant improvement ($p<0.01$) in VABS-II communication raw score and total adaptive score
- ✓ VABS-II communication improvements significant for expressive language (pre: 82.7; post: 89.4; $p < 0.01$), but not receptive language ($p = 0.06$, n.s.)
- ✓ ANCOVA compared waitlist control to THR and found significant improvement in ABC-C Irritability, Hyperactivity, Lethargy and Stereotype subscales ($p<0.01$)

Both of the researches show that hippotherapy and Therapeutic Horseback riding can and are effective tools of intervention for children and youth with ASD. As the EAAT field grows more research is needed on its effects on ASD population including adults.

So now that we know that EAAT can be a successful, fun, and effective activity for ASD population let us focus on some practical aspects of this industry.

CHAPTER FOURTEEN

How To Choose A Good Riding Center

So hopefully you decided that EAATs are for your family. Now comes the very important part. How to make sure, that we are putting our children or ourselves in safe hands. There are a few things that can help us decide which center is a best fit for you.

First and for most the place has to be safe!!!!!! If you have ever worked with horses before the decision process will be much easier, but if this is your first contact with equines, no problem, here are few things to look out for.

1. The safest bet is an accredited center or at least accredited instructor

Most countries have organizations that govern EAAT activities and certifications. In the USA PATH International is one of the major organizations that certifies both centers and instructors. In Poland this role lies in the hands of Polish Hippotherapy Association. Germany has different organizations governing different areas of EAAT's. Check your local resources for the information on your country.

PATH Int. has different levels of accreditations for centers. A center can be a member, which promises to uphold to standards, or it can become a Premier Accredited Center. This means that the center went through a very strict accreditation process and was evaluated by an evaluation committee in different areas such as: written procedures and policies, quality and safety of horse care and horse management, volunteer training, risk management and more. These centers are reevaluated every five years. Choosing a center with this type of accreditation is the safest way to go.

Second safety check is the certification of the instructor. PATH International provides three levels of therapeutic riding instructor certifications: registered, advanced and master. Most instructor hold the registered certification which is sufficient for the purpose of safety. To be certified as a registered instructor one has to pass an on line exam, complete internship, and pass a practical riding and teaching exam. After obtaining certification, all instructors have to complete 20 hours of continued education each year and be current on First aid and CPR certifications for both adult and children.

There is also a special certification for each type of EAAT activity besides riding. Right now, PATH International provides certification in driving, vaulting, Equine Specialist in Mental Health and Learning. There is also a separate organization called American Hippotherapy Association that provides certification for hippotherapy. Yet another organization, Certified Horsemanship Association (CHA), provides very good standards in able-body instructor certification and center certification. It also has a certification for therapeutic horseback riding instructors, which is mostly based on PATH International standards. Another organization that provides standards for Equine Assisted Psychotherapy and Equine Assisted Learning is The Equine Assisted Growth and Learning Association (EAGALA) . This organization supports a team model. The teams consist of an equine specialist and a license clinician.

It is important to note that in USA there is no legal obligation to be certified as a riding instructor (other than state of Massachusetts) or to be certified as a therapeutic instructor if one is providing recreational/sport riding lessons. One has to be licensed in a given state as a therapist to provide occupational, speech, or physical therapy. Making sure that your provider is certified is a very important for your safety. Also check your country's laws and certifications that an instructor may be required to obtain.

2. **Make sure that your provider is familiar with your diagnosis.**

Next step in the process of choosing a safe place is to meet in person with your future instructor and discus your current situation, your approach and your needs. Premier PATH centers will have an initial evaluation procedure in place. This is the time when you don't see the horses but get to know your future provider. Don't be afraid to ask any questions and make sure that you answer truthfully to the questions from the staff. Hiding anything just to make sure that you will have a place to ride is not a good idea and puts you and other participants of the program in danger. It may also lead to frustration on both sides. Not all centers are equipped to handle every client and sometimes it is better to look for a different option. On the other hand if the instructors are not sure or cannot answer some of your questions it may not be a good match either.

You will be asked about things like weight and height. This part is important in the process of matching a horse to the rider. Weight limits are in place for the well-being of our four legged friends who work very hard in the centers. The general rule is that rider should not weight more than 20% of the horse's body mass, but it is up to the stuff to decide which horse is going to suit the needs of the client best.

You will also be asked to fill out forms about medical history and receive doctor's permission. This is important, because there are medical and psychological contraindications to horseback riding. Remember that if you or your child is not able to participate in horseback riding lesson you may still take part in driving or unmounted activities like brushing.

3. Use your common sense and judgment!!!!

If something doesn't seem right, the place makes you uncomfortable or you are not satisfied with the state of equipment, horses, or instruction, discuss it with your provider! If you are still not at ease, move on. Make sure that you or your child always rides or drives in a helmet. Look around. Is the place clean and neat? Is there farm equipment with sharp edges lying around? Is the manure cleaned on a regular basis? Is the horse tack (equipment) in good condition? Are the horses calm and in good health or can you see them limping and bones sticking out? Is the arena that you are riding in enclosed? Are the personnel polite? During the lesson is the riding space calm and safe? This is your time and you should enjoy it. So use your judgment and listen to your "gut feeling".

So what should you expect?

So you chose a safe place to ride...What's next?....Well it depends on the center and on the type of EAAT but let's look at the most likely scenario with therapeutic horseback riding.

After your evaluation session, which was briefly described above, you will be invited for your first riding session. You will probably have an assigned volunteer or a staff member that will help you with getting your helmet. If part of your lesson involves cleaning and tacking up your horse, you will also get assistance with obtaining the proper equipment or someone will get it for you. You may also ride in a center where your horse is waiting ready for you. And you may be asked to buy your own helmet. Remember that wearing appropriate clothes is very important for safety and comfort. You should always have long pants on, and if riding in a saddle, boots with higher heal. Also the stirrups should have a safety mechanism so that in case of a fall your leg will not get stuck. Your instructor should advise you on the proper equipment that is appropriate for your activity.

Once you and the horse are ready you will be escorted to the mounting area. This is the place where you get on the horse. There are several methods of getting on the horse. The two most common in a therapeutic setting are mounting block and the ramp. The staff should explain the procedure and guide you through getting on the horse. Before mounting the horse your instructor or a trained volunteer should check one more time that all the equipment on the horse is properly fitting. Most importantly if the girth (the part of tack that holds your saddle or surcingle to the horse and goes underneath its belly) is tight. Once you are on the horse the stirrups will be adjusted.

After you enter the arena the gate or door to the riding ring should be closed. You can also go on trail rides and on sensory trails. In that case there will be no enclosure. Depending on your level of riding ability and needs you may have an assigned leader and or side walker. The first part of the lesson usually consists of warm ups which are simple exercise (ex arm circles). Next is the lesson itself. At the end the instructor will review the skills that you learned, your accomplishments and you will be asked to dismount the horse. The instructor or volunteers will escort you to the barn, and instruct you to either help with putting the horse away or finish your lesson.

This of course is a very basic scenario and it can differ from barn to barn and even instructor to instructor. The main part of the lesson will depend on your skill level, abilities and goals.

Next I will present some possible exercises and activities that may help in more difficult situations.

CHAPTER FIFTEEN

What To Do If......

In this section I would like to present some options and activities, re-actions and exercises that may come in handy in situations that are not so typical. First let's talk about the "elephant in the room": difficult behaviors during activities on, and around the horse.

DIFFICULT BEHAVIORS

What are difficult behaviors? Those are behaviors that are challeng-ing, inappropriate at the moment or socially unacceptable. They can occur in any age group and have many reasons. They create prob-lems for the participant themselves and for people around them. These are situations that if a client is ask to stop doing something they continue to do the behavior or escalate the behavior. In a EAAT set-ting they can be quiet unsafe and should not be left unnoticed. It is worth mentioning that a single incident of difficult behavior, if dealt with inappropriately, may lead to future occurrences of the same be-havior. Each event involving difficult behavior should be analyzed by the instructor or therapist. In case of a group lesson or if client pre-sents lots of undesirable behavior the lead instructor should ask for help and allow someone else from the team to observe the session. Another therapeutic approach in analyzing the situation is video- re-cording. Sometimes we may find out that something that we thought is purely behavioral may be related to sensory problems or based on physical issues.

Here are the examples of most common difficult behaviors:

Tantrum tantrum-

"A tantrum(or temper tantrum or tirade or hissy fit) is an emotional outburst, usually associated with children or those in emotional dis-tress, it is typically characterized by stubbornness, crying, screaming, yelling, shrieking, defiance, angry ranting, a resistance to attempts at pacification and, in some cases, violence" . We all have experience a tantrum from a child at least once in our life time. A good example of this during a horseback riding activity will be a child who likes to trot and wants to trot all the time. When a different exercise is introduce he or she will scream "No, I want to trot" and may proceed to kick the horse or refuse to participate in anything other than trotting. So what should we do? Ignoring the behavior can lead to a dangerous situation. A wrong reaction can lead to even more problems. So what's the solution? Using the ABC method described in the earlier part of this book (in the section about ABA therapy) we can analyze the situation. Does the child like to trot because it seeks vestibular stimulation? Are we providing exercises and activities that are appropriate for his or her age and the activities are engaging? Are the choices given interesting for the client? Do we follow through with our promises and comments? Do we set up clear boundaries? If we rearward the kicking and screaming with a trot...we can be pretty sure that the situation will repeat itself. A best solution would be a calm response along the lines of: "You will get to trot after we finish warm up exercises. We will reach to the horse's ears and then you can trot for 10 strides." If a clear and calm response does not bring any effects, we may be force to introduce a stronger reaction. My strongest reaction in this type of situation is to dismount the client. Usually I make the consequences very clear at the beginning of a behavior. Here is a twist...We have to be absolutely sure that we can follow through with the consequence. There is nothing worse than not following through when the client decides to test how serious we are about what we say. So if for example I was on a trail ride with a client who uses a wheelchair and weights almost as much as I do, and there is no easy way of getting him or her back to the barn other than on horseback, a threat of dismount would not be a best idea . A dismount would also be my last resort in most situations. The first step would be a choice (if you do A we will do B). Second would be a set-up of time frame with a count- down to a consequence (John, your behavior right now is dangerous, please stop. I will count down to 10 and if you cannot calm yourself down, you will have to walk back to the barn next to the horse). Then begin the countdown...if I get to three (which seldom happens) I will remind them about the consequence and then follow through with it. In my experience, if a behavior is a result of a tantrum tentrum, usually following through once or twice teaches the client that there is a no "win" for him once the countdown begins.

Sexual behaviors

Working with diverse age groups you will sooner or later run into a problem of inappropriate sexual behaviors. These behaviors can have different forms. Masturbation during the ride, inappropriate touching of volunteers or other staff members, talking about sexual encounters or fantasies these are all examples of inappropriate sexual behaviors.

So how do we deal with this type of behavior? As usual, prevention is our best first choice. Identifying the "why" behind a given behavior may allow us to prevent it in a future. Things to avoid in the case of clients with inappropriate tendencies include hugging, arm over leg side walking, sitting trot, and hands on postural corrections. We may also discover that our clients "fall in love" with some of the volunteers. A larger center can provide a better choice of volunteers and instructors (for example, a man for heterosexual male client). If the clients mental capacity allows for understanding the topic, we may explain why a given behaviors is not appropriate. Therapist and caregivers should also understand that none of the team members (including the instructors) should be put in a position that they have to deal with something that they are not comfortable with. If the sexual behaviors cannot be controlled and creates a serious problem, the center may be forced to discontinue its services for a given client.

Use of inappropriate language

Inappropriate language, although by itself not dangerous, can negatively influence other participants and staff members and is socially unacceptable. It can be caused by a few factors. Seeking attention, emotional regulation (tension release) and inability to correctly express ones needs and wants are among the most common causes of this behavior. Of course depending on the cause, our reaction should be different. Working one on one and avoiding group situations should be our priority. Identifying the roots of the problems and praising the appropriate behavior while ignoring the inappropriate language may also prove effective.

Physical aggression towards therapist, horse or staff

Physical aggression should never be tolerated and should be immediately stopped. If this type of behavior reoccurs and cannot be controlled a dismissal from the program may be appropriate. Aggression can include hitting, biting, scratching, hair pulling, punching, kicking, spiting. Depending on the clients' size and strength it may be gentle or strong. No matter the clients strength this type of behavior cannot be tolerated. One needs to remember that small children become big adults and if such behavior continues it may put staff and other participants in serious danger. Although very often the root of the behavior cannot be identified, the most common reasons include: inability to communicate properly (especially in the case of nonverbal clients), emotional regulation, being afraid, and reaction to stimuli (oversensitivity).

So what to do if the behavior occurs? The instructor or therapist should calmly stop the behavior and if necessary dismount and move to a different activity. The safety of everyone involved (including the horse) should be the top priority. If the cause of behavior cannot be identify and the behavior reoccurs and poses a danger the dismissal from the program may be necessary.

Behaviors that put the client at risk

Behaviors such as falling of the horse on purpose or slowly sliding to the side are very dangerous and should not be tolerated. The most common reasons for falling off or jumping off on purpose are problems with prioprioception and sensory integration. This kind of problem can be solved by providing exercises that in a safe way stimulate these senses. For example "Over the barrel " position or sitting trot at the beginning of the lesson should help to minimize the occurrence of this type of behavior.

Slow sliding to the side but not falling all together can be an example of provocation and testing the boundaries. The client usually makes sure that he/she is being closely watched and supervised and repeats the behavior with a smile or laugh knowing that it is forbidden. Setting up unpleasant consequence (like an exercise that the client doesn't like after each attempt) usually solves this pattern of behavior.

Constantly asking the same question over and over

Asking the same question over and over can most commonly be caused by three different reasons:

1.   Echolalia. Some clients living with ASD have a echolalia which is automotive repetition of sounds made by the other person but it also can present itself in constant repetition of the same phrases or asking over and over the same questions. Controlling echolalia is a very difficult task since it is base in neurobiology. During therapeutic horseback riding sessions the goal is to minimize the influence of this behavior on the activity at hand. Some clients may respond well to ignoring the question after it was answered the first time, if we are sure that the client knows the answer. Others may do better if we ask the question back or talk about a different topic. Yet another person may want to hear the answer over and over. Also with higher function-ing clients setting a time to answer questions may prove effective.

2.   Asking the same questions do to anxiety or anticipation. Some client may ask a series of questions pertaining to what will fol-low, or how much time is left, or which horse is being used etc. These questions very often arise from anxiety and fear. This type of ques-tions should be treated very seriously and be answered each time be-cause they provide a security blanket to the client.

3.   Asking the questions as an avoidance/reward mecha-nism. In this situation the most common question that I hear is "can we trot now?" They may also be trying to push for a favorite exercise, or, for not doing an exercise that is least favored but very important for skill building. I find that in this type of situations having a board with a lesson schedule or clearly stating what is next usually solves the prob-lem.

EMOTION EXPRESSION, IDENTIFICATION AND REGULATION

A lot of people on the ASD spectrum are not aware of their emotions and do not identify the varying degrees of emotions. They may also require help with identification of the physical sensation of emotions and coaching on appropriate expression and regulation of their feelings. The EAAT setting is a perfect place to bring attention to emotions and feelings of the clients and others around him/her.

Bringing awareness to one's body and engaging in communication about what the horse, therapist and volunteers may feel in a given situation may help. For example if a client always expresses anger in an extreme manor. He or she does not distinguish between being "very mad" and "slightly mad". He/she also may not be able to tell how his/hers body feels in these different situations and what emotion is attached to a given "feel". Identifying the level of anger or happiness on a visual scale and bringing attention to the bodies feelings associated with it may allow the client to better understanding his or her emotional world and to prevent uncontrollable outbursts. Once a client knows "how anger feels" ahead of time he or she may remove him/herself out of a given situation or ask for help. At that point relaxation exercises and breathing techniques may also be introduced to help them deal with anger and anxiety.

Being aware of ones emotional state opens the door to learning how to correctly express a given emotion. Happiness, anger, anxiety can all be expressed in socially acceptable or unacceptable ways. Once a client learns the more acceptable way of emotional expression his chances of forming meaningful relationships increase.

BEING ABLE TO CHANGE ROUTINE

A lot of autistic children have various degrees of difficulties in changing the routine. Some parents report problems so severe that it is very difficult to introduce even the smallest change in the daily routine. For example a slight change in the bus route due to the road construction, can cause tremendous tantrums and put the child off balance for the rest of the day. In my experience the child that exhibits high anxiety due to a routine change benefits from slow introduction of anything new. The more exposure to new situations the bigger likelihood of lowering anxiety in the next new situation. This system works, of course, only if we are careful not to traumatize the child by introducing to many things too fast.

In the context of EAATs there are two aspects of change that I feel need addressing:

- ✓ introduction of EAAT to child's routine
- ✓ changes of the EAAT routine itself.

Challenges of Introducing EAAT

Starting therapeutic horseback riding lessons or hippotherapy can be challenging for any person. We are interacting with animals that usually are a lot bigger than ourselves and as live animals sometimes are slightly unpredictable. Horses can move when not asked, make noises and they smell differently. The barn is a totally new place that does not resemble anything that we have been exposed to before, and it has its own set of rules. Introduction to EAAT can be somewhat challenging for anyone let alone a child that already doesn't like any changes in the routine.

In my 12 years of work with the ASD population and horses I have come across a few clients that initially were deemed "impossible to put on a horse". Out of all of these clients only one did not finally get on a horse with a smile on his or her face. All of the above clients required "creative" approaches. Here are some of the "the tricks" that I use in this type of situations:

- ➢ Schedule the last lesson of a day (or only lesson of a day) and don't set a time limit on the lesson. On some days it may be 10 minutes on others 2 hr (my personal record was 4 hr.)
- ➢ Start without horses. Introduce the facilities and allow client to watch activities. Slowly start introducing familiar activities (as throwing a ball) in the barn or near horses or just on the new grounds near the client's car.

Introduce the horse as an "incident" For example...have the volunteer walk the horse next to the area that you play...and role the ball towards the horse (of course the horse has to be desensitize to balls and don't through the ball to close to the animal) or walk the horse through the aisle that the child is standing in.

- ➢ If possible start with brushing and touching the horse....if not...try taking the horse for a "Leash walk"
- ➢ If the child at any moment wants to leave, let it do so, with supervision.

➤ Sometimes the group approach works better....the child would like to join other children...or mimic adults...but with ASD that may be a bit tricky.

➤ Start the activity that you want the child to participate in and overly exaggerate "the fun" you are having. Note that you really have to have fun. Children pick up really easily on our true "feelings".

➤ Picture boards and schedules are also very handy tools.

➤ Be creative...sometimes the most unconventional ideas are the best.

➤ Plan ahead but don't be upset if nothing goes according to the plan.

BE VERY VERY PATIENT.....it may take a few weeks or a year....

Challenges of change in the EAAT routine

Working with and around horses can pose some challenges. In EAAT our main therapeutic tool is life, breathing and feeling organism. Sometimes our horses get sick, sometimes they have a not so good day and sometimes we have to make sure that they are not working to much (the same applies to volunteers and other staff members). The most common issues with EAAT routines that I have encountered so far are:

✓ Having to change a horse;
✓ Having to change members of the group lesson;
✓ Having to change the barn routine;
✓ Having to change volunteers.

As you can see most of the events may or may not be unexpected. It is easier to deal with transitions if we can prepare for them. One way of doing so is by writing things down for the parents and participants so that they review coming changes between the session. Also if it possible a slow, gradual transition will always be easier than a rapid one. For example, if the instructor feels that the child is outgrowing a pony/horse he or she may slowly introduce the new animal by first talking about the other horse, having someone else riding it in the presence of the client, visiting the new horse in the pasture/ stall just to say hi, then grooming and comparing the similarities between the two animals and finally having a "try" lesson on the new mount. In my experience that usually leads to a successful transition.

The situation becomes a bit more complicated if the change is unexpected. Life happens and sometimes we need to adapt quickly. A lot of our clients are not very good at handling "surprises". I found that being open about the change and going through steps similar to the ones described above may lessen the impact of unexpected change. If a horse gets sick or loses a shoe we may talk to the client about similar situations that they have been in and about the fact that they may make "new friends" with another horse. In the case of clients with severe anxiety we may have to take few steps back and basically restart the whole process of getting them acquainted with a new team member. If we know that the client will be extremely anxious or the transition will not be successful in the case of a single lesson we may be better off canceling that session. That said, I like to change horses and staff members for each clients on regular basis and without reason just because it sets a "norm" for not expecting the given horse or given staff. That makes the unexpected life situations so much easier. It also has an added benefit: clients learning to better handle changes in other situations.

Another important factor in changing anything in the lesson routine is making it seem as "normal" and casual as possible or even better, presenting the change as an exciting and interesting new opportunity. This technique is only successful if our own feelings about the transition are genuine. If we will try "faking it" most of the clients will pick up on it and we may end up losing trust and setting ourselves for an interesting lesson time.

PHYSICAL DEVELOPMENT- WHICH EXERCISE WHEN AND WHY

Physical development is the act or process of natural progression in physical maturation (as distinguished from the mind). It usually refers to the time from birth till physical maturity, although some components of physical characteristic can (and should) be developed throughout the life span.

Growing children undergo changes in all the body systems. Their bones are growing and so do the cardiovascular and pulmonary systems both increasing their capacity and also becoming more efficient. The muscles are increasing their mass, their blood supply increases and they become faster. The bones grow, and become stronger. The brain and nervous system undergo the most severe and complicated changes. All of them allow for motor development. The developing brain enables physical coordination. As the muscle and nervous system mature more complicated motor skills emerge.

As mentioned in Part II of this book motor skills development is essential to the progression of life skills. Motor development includes balance, general coordination, eye hand coordination, body awareness and spatial orientation, muscle strength, and last but not least manual dexterity. All of these components translate to the ability to cope and execute daily living activities. Let's look at ways that we can influence the development of each through EAAT.

Balance

Horseback riding and general barn activities are a very good means for balance development. Just passively sitting on a moving horse requires constant balance readjustment. Walking around the barn also requires working on somewhat uneven terrain as is stepping on the mounting block and mounting ramp. The biggest balance benefits however can always be gained by mounted activities where the horse provides a constant unstable, elevated base of support.

The most basic balance exercise starts with the correct sitting position while facing forward. After achieving this position at a standstill we can introduce walk. As mentioned before (LOOK UP PAGE NUMBER) the constant change of a horse's center of gravity forces the rider to change their center of gravity. The same can be said about moving the rider's different parts of the body. It is also worth mentioning that riding in a saddle requires less balance than riding with surcingle.

As with any exercise it is important to keep in mind the progression of difficulty. The first step up from basic forward facing position will be accomplished by different hands/arm positions. Here is the progression of difficulty for facing forward:

➢ Facing forward hand on front saddle pummel/ or surcingle

- Facing forward hand on rider's thighs
- Facing forward hand on rider's hips
- Facing forward hand resting behind the rider
- Facing forward with rider's hands under his/her buttocks
- Facing forward arms to the side
- Facing forward arms above the head
- Facing forward trunk rotations with arm to the side
- Facing forward reaching for the horses' ears and tail.
- Facing forward and reaching to different parts of the body of both horse and the rider or side walker.

It is very important that the rider sustains a correct pelvic position during these exercises.

The next level of progression for balance exercises involves changing the seat position on the horses. These are the exercises that usually are done without a saddle and come from a vaulting background. They include:

- Sitting backwards (facing the tail of the horse).
- Sitting sideways (remember to spend equal amount of time on both sides unless the goals are to even out muscle imbalance)
- "Around the world" exercise (also known as "Mary go around") where rider actively changes position with or without help from forward sitting to sideway to facing the tail to sideways back to forward sitting.
- Kneeling on the horse with the hands resting on the horse.
- Kneeling on the horse with the arms stretched out to the side.

If the center has access to a well-trained vaulting horse and vaulting instructor the ultimate and most difficult position is standing up on the horse.

All of the above progressions can be achieved at standstill or walk. For the more advance riders most of them can be achieved in trot. In the case of advanced vaulting sessions they can also be tried at center.

Motor coordination

Motor coordination is the ability to control and direct different body parts to execute complicate intended movements in a smooth, efficient and well timed way. The simplest division of coordination refers to gross motor skills and fine motors skills. The gross motor skills address movement such as jumping, playing drums, or throwing a ball. Fine motor skills address precise actions such as writing, threading beads and cutting with scissors. Besides this most basic division we can also talk about other types of motor coordination. The most prominent is hand –eye coordination that relates to an ability to coordinate the eye movement with hand movement. Worth addressing is also bilateral coordination which refers to the ability to use both sides of the body in a coordinated way. It also relates to spatial orientation,

Gross motor skills and EAAT

Riding a horse in itself requires a lot of gross motor skills. Changing gates, staying in balance with a horse's motion and at the same time controlling the horse's direction and speed all require a lot of motor skills. Learning how to post during trot or how to assume a jumping position (also known as two point of half seat) requires a lot of gross motor skills. For more advance riders canter can be introduced. The rider also needs to be able to react to different situations and obstacles.

If our clients need more work on gross motor skills we can introduce a series of beneficial exercises. Riding in a circle or completing a slalom is the simplest form of coordination and balance challenge other than riding a straight line. We can also develop different obstacle courses that introduce different stations like going over jumping poles, catching a ball, reaching for things that hang of the wall and moving things from one point of the ring to another. Going on a trail ride that includes hills is also a very good way to incorporate gross motor skills into the lesson theme. For more advance riders we can introduce small jumps or going under tree branches. Of course the horses use for such lessons have to be previously introduced to the obstacles and equipment used so that everyone is safe.

Muscle strength and EAAT

Horseback riding and barn work by themselves are a great way to develop muscle strength. If you ever had a chance to ride a horse you know that it's definitely a lot more physical work than it looks. When I had my own practice in Poland I had a rule that at least one parent of each of my clients had to get on a horse for at least 15 minutes. All of the core muscle and major muscles in the arms and legs get a good workout just by simple riding in the correct position at walk and trot. During therapy session we can also introduce additional exercises which target different muscle groups. Depending on the comfort level of the instructor or therapist and the knowledge of personal training one can introduce some elements of yoga and strength training including exercise with resistance bands and resistance against the body of the instructor.

Hand –eye coordination in EAAT

Hand-eye coordination is the ability of the vision system to coordinate the received information to control, guide, and direct the hands to achieve a given task, such as handwriting or catching a ball . Hand - eye coordination uses the eyes to direct attention and the hands to execute a task. We can measure the efficiency of this coordination by comparing how fast and precise one can manipulate different objects, and how precisely one can throw.

Hand eye coordination can be practiced during mounted and unmounted activities.

Grooming a horse, with the focus on precision, putting away equipment, reaching for different brushes can all be incorporated to an unmounted session.

During riding lessons or hippotherapy sessions we incorporate exercises such us:

- ➢ Touching different parts of the horses body
- ➢ Throwing a ball into different targets that can be placed at different heights and distances,
- ➢ Picking toys off the walls and stations

> Moving toys and equipment from one place to another
> Placing rings on different sticks or arms of volunteers
> Throwing and catching the ball above ones head
> Throwing and catching the ball to and from side walker/instructor
> Bouncing the ball from the wall

One can also raise the level of difficulty by combining activities like throwing the ball, touching a given part of horse and catching the ball or during a group lesson passing the ball/object to a classmate. The combinations and creativity are limited only by safety and a student's ability. It is very important to remember that the horse should be tested for each piece of equipment/ exercise before the game can be introduced during lesson.

Body awareness and spatial orientation

Body awareness refers to how the body senses itself. How do you know if you are hungry or cold? How do you know if your arm is moving? There are three different pathways that allow our body to build knowledge about itself:

1. Prioprioception-which referees to the body's awareness of movements and behaviors. When you close your eyes how do you know where your feet, hands and ears are? How do you know if your arm is bent or straight? There are two parts to prioprioception. First one is kinesthesia, which is the awareness of the position and movement of the parts of the body using sensory organs, which are known as proprioceptors, in joints and muscles. Second part is balance which originates in the inner ear.

2. Interception- is how we perceive pain hunger and movement of internal organ (such as lungs);

3. Exteroception -is how we perceive the outside world. It contains all our senses. It is the information from the skin, smell, taste, vision and hearing receptors.

Since we do not live in a vacuum the body awareness is always connected to the spatial orientation, which is the ability to maintain our body orientation and/or posture in relation to the surrounding environment (physical space) at rest and during motion. It relies on the use of visual, vestibular, and proprioceptive receptors that send sensory information. Changes in linear acceleration, angular acceleration, and gravity are detected by the vestibular system and the proprioceptive receptors, and then compared in the brain with visual information.

The development of both body awareness and spatial orientation depends on the quantity and quality of the movement one has experienced since birth. The more we move, the more varied experience we have the bigger chances of developing correct body awareness and better spatial orientation. EAAT gives us a unique opportunity to experience our body in three dimensional movements, and to build better awareness of such body parts as knees, hips, trunk and also previously discussed balance.

Here are some examples of exercise that can increase the awareness of body parts:

Knees:

> Holding a piece of paper between the knees and saddle or knees and the horse
> Posting trot with and without stirrups
> Touching knee to elbow on the same side of the body
> Touching knee to elbow on the diagonal
> Bouncing the ball on the knee

Hips:

> Walk or trot with hands on the hips
> "Pushing the horse forward" at walk or trot
> Sitting trot
> "Around the word"
> For more advance riders jumping position and center

Trunk:

> Trunk rotations with arms to the side
> Dismount through turning to the stomach

> Lying prone on horses back while facing forward (must be done without saddle) can be done at walk and stand still
> Laying on the stomach and reaching the tail while facing backwards
> Hugging the horse's neck while facing forward
> Touching a horses ears while laying on the neck
> Laying prone across the horses body

Feet:

> Putting weight on the stirrup
> Standing up in the stirrups
> Circles with the feet
> Holding a ring on the tip of the boot while riding from one point to another
> Standing on tip toes in the stirrup (make sure side-walkers are available)

If our clients have difficulty with naming body parts or difficulties with spatial relations we can introduce games that include touching different body parts of the horse or volunteer   Building obstacles courses and going "under" or "around" can be also very helpful in strengthening spatial skills. "Simon says" is a perfect game to introduce these type of skills.

Bilateral coordination

Bilateral coordination is the ability to use both sides of the body at the same time. It refers to using the two sides for the same action (like using a rolling pin) or using alternating movements (like climbing stairs). Bilateral coordination is also required for using each side of your body for a different action, such as holding food with the fork and at the same time cutting with the knife. It is important because it allows both sides of the body to work in a smooth and fluid motion.

Any symmetrical mounted activities at walk and trot at straight line will stimulate the bilateral coordination. The three dimensional symmetrical movement of the horse forces the rider to use his or her body equally. We can also stimulate bilateral coordination by emphasizing equal work in both direction and symmetrical exercises. For example if we ask the student to do one exercise with the right hand we should give him or her equal opportunity and encourage him or her to do the same with the opposite hand.

It is important to note that riding in a circle both for the horse and the rider creates asymmetry. The same can be said about canter work for more advance students.

For me one of the most important skills that relies on bilateral coordination is crossing the midline of the body. We cross the midline each time we put a part of our body in the space of the one on the opposite side. For example, touching the right shoulder with the left hand or sitting cross legged both require crossing the midline.

Besides developing bilateral coordination and body awareness all exercises that require crossing the midline have an additional positive effect: they synchronize the work of right brain hemisphere with the left brain hemisphere. They also bring better awareness to both sides of the body and emphasize using both sides of the body equally. Here are some examples of exercise during mounted and unmounted EAAT activities.

Unmounted:

- ➢ Brushing the horse with both hands holding the brush
- ➢ Brushing the horse with one hand in one direction and the other hand in the other direction
- ➢ Brushing the horse with one hand and then switching the brush to the other hand
- ➢ Holding the brush in the hand that is closer to the horse and curry comb in the other. Between each circular brushing motion of the horse the student cleans the brush on the curry comb.
- ➢ Independently picking and cleaning all four hoofs.
- ➢ Tack cleaning
- ➢ Pushing the a wheel -barrel with both hands
- ➢ Carrying a saddle in front of the body with both hands
- ➢ Reaching for equipment with both hands.

Mounted:

Symmetrical:

> ➤ Both hand touch the horses ears at the same time
> ➤ Arms circle forward and backwards
> ➤ Facing backwards touching the horses tail with both hands
> ➤ Holding back pommel clapping both feet over horses neck
> ➤ Touching both knees over the front pommel
> ➤ Grabbing an object with both hands and while rotating passing it to a person on the other side.

Asymmetrical:

> ➤ Arm circles: one arm forward one arm backward at the same time
> ➤ Touching one knee to elbow at the same side of the body
> ➤ Touching different parts of the leg with the hand at the same side of the body
> ➤ Riding in a circle
> ➤ Picking a correct lead in center for more advance riders.

Crossing the midline

> ➤ Right hand touches the left ear of the horse
> ➤ Right hand puts a ring on the left foot
> ➤ Grab a ring from a side-walker on the left side of the horse with your left hand and put it on the right horses ear (or give it to the side walker on the right)
> ➤ Pick up a ball from the string on the wall with your left hand, trot right, and while keeping the ball in the left hand put it in a basket on the right.
> ➤ Right elbow touches left knee

Manual dexterity

Manual dexterity refers to fine motor skills of hands and fingers. Fine motors skill is the coordination of muscle, bones, and nerves to produce small, precise movements which occur in different body parts usually in coordination with the eyes. Development of manual dexterity is necessary for development of independent daily living skills.

Working with and around horses creates lots of opportunity to develop manual dexterity. Holding the rains, brushing the horse, cleaning the tack, buckling and unbuckling different parts of a bridle, helping around the barn, tacking up all by themselves all help to develop small motor skills. Additionally during the riding lesson we can include games and exercises that develop those skills even more. Here are some examples:

> ➤ Squishing different balls with one or both hands. The balls can be hard or spongy or made out of jell.
> ➤ Picking small objects out of a bag
> ➤ Rolling a small ball on the horses back while facing backwards
> ➤ Clipping and unclipping laundry clips (or hair clips) to the horses main.
> ➤ Braiding the horses main and tail
> ➤ Walking the fingers on the horses neck up to its ears
> ➤ Touching fingers to each other in a different order
> ➤ Patting the horse
> ➤ Grabbing rings on an obstacle course
> ➤ Rolling up bandages

LITERATURE:

Bauman, M.,L., Kemper, T., I. (1994) Neuroanatomical observations of the brain in autism. In: Bauman, M., L. Kemper T., L. red (2006) *The Neurobiology of Autism.* The Johns Hopkins University Press: Baltimore.

Benda, W., McGibbon, N.H, Grant, K.L. (2003). Improvements in muscle symmetry in children with cerebral palsy after equine-assisted therapy (hippotherapy). *The Journal of Alternative and Complementary Medicine*, 9, 817-825.

Berkson, (1996). Feedback and control in the development of abnormal stereotyped behaviors. In R. Sprague & K. Newell (Eds.) *Stereotyped movements: Brain and behavior relationships* (pp. 3-15). Washington, DC: APA.

Biery M.J. , (1985) Riding and the handicapped. *Vet Clin North Am Small Anim Pract.* 15, p. 345-354.

Bobkowicz-Lewartowska, L. (2005). *Autyzm dziecięcy: zagadnienia diagnoza i terapia.* Oficyna Wydawnicza Impuls, Kraków.

Brauner A. F.,(1993). *Dziecko zagubione w rzeczywistości.* Wydawnictwa Szkolne i Pedagogiczne, Warszawa

Clark M., Plante E. (1998) Morphology of the inferior frontal gyrus in developmentally language disordered adults. *Brain Language* 61: 288-303

Clayton, H.M. (2004). *The dynamic horse. A biomechainical guide to equine movement and performance.* Mason, MI: Sport Horse Publications

Courchesne, E., Townsend J., Saitoh O. (1994). The brain in infantile autism: Posterior fossa structures are abnormal. *Neurology* 44: 214-223.

De Fosse, Hodge S., Harris G, et al. (2002). An abnormal volumetric asymmetry pattern in language processing cortical areas in children with autism and children with SLI. *Presented at the conference: International Meeting for Autism Research*, Orlando, Fla., November 1-2

Delacato C. H., (1995) *Dziwne, niepojętne. Autystyczne Dziecko.* Fundacja Synapsis, Warszawa

Dunn L.S., Donaldson C. (2001). Integration of the Sensorimotor Approach within the Classroom. W : Huebner, R. (2001). *Autism: a sensory motor approach.* S:297-311 Maryland: Aspen Publishers' Inc.

Dunn W. (1994) Performance of Typical Children on the Sensory Profile: An Item Analysis. *The American Journal of Occupational Therapy 48 (11)"* 967-974

Fisher A.G., Murray, E.A. (1991) Introduction to sensory integration theory. In Fisher A.G. Murray, E. A., Bundy A.C. (red.). *Sensoryintegration theory and practice* (p. 3-26). Filadelfia :F.A. Davis.

Fix J. (1997) *Neuroanatomia.* Urban & Partner. Wydawnictwo Medyczne Wrocław.

Gillberg C. (1992) Subgroups in autism: are there behavioural phenotypes typical of underlying medical conditions? *J Intell Disab Res 36:201-14.*

Gliman, S. Newman, S.W. (1992) *Essentials of Clinical neuroanatomy and neurophysiology* (8ed) Philadelphia: F.A. Davis.

Grabowski, J. (1982) *Hipologia dla wszystkich.* Warsaw: Krajowa Agencja Wydawnicza,

Harris, Susan E. ,(1993) *Horse Gait, Balance and Movement.* New York: Howell Book House 1993 p. 42-44

Guess, D., & Carr, E. (1991). Emergence and maintenance of stereo-typy and self-injury. *American Journal on Mental Retardation*, 96, 299-319

Gutstein S. (2009). *The RDI Book: Forging New Pathways for Autsim, Asperger's and PDD with the Relationship Development Inter-vention Program.* Houston: Connection Center Publishing.

Hachl V. et al. (1999) The influence of Hippotherapy on the Kinemat-ics and Functional Performance of Two Children with Cerebral Palsy. *Pediatric Physical Therapy* 11, 89-101.

Happe, F., (1994). *Autism: an introduction to psychological theory.* Harvard University Press, Cambridge Massachusetts.

Hass, R. H., Townsend, J. Courchesne, E., Lincoln,. A. J., Schreib-man, L., i Yeung-Courchesne R. (1996) Neurological abnormali-ties in infantile autism. *Journal of Child Neurology*, 11, 84-92.

Herbert MR, Harris GJ, Adrien Kt, et al. (2002). Abnormal asymmetry in language association cortex in autism. *Annals of Neurology* 52: 588-96.

Huebner and Lane (2001). Neuropsychological Findings, Etiology, and Implications for Autism. In: Huebner, R. (2001). *Autism: a senso-ry motor approach.* Maryland: Aspen Publishers' Inc.

Huebner, R.A., Dunn, W., (2001) Introduction and Basic Concepts. In: Huebner, R. (2001*). Autism: a sensory motor approach.* Mary-land: Aspen Publishers' Inc.

Jones V., Prior M. (1985). Motor Imitation Abilities and Neurological Signs in Autistic Children. *Journal of Autism and Developmental Disorders*, 5: 37-45.

Kemner C. , C., Verbaten, M. N., Cuperus, J. M., Camfferman, G. & van Engeland, H (1998). Abnormal Saccadic Eye Movements in Autistic Children. *Journal of Autism and Developmental Disor-ders* 28(1): 61-67

Kohen-Raz R., Volkmar F, R., Cohen D. J (1992) Postural Control in Children with Autism. *Journal of Autism and Developmental Disorders* 22(3): 419-432

Kwolek, A. Ed. (2003). *Rehabilitacja medyczna Tom II*. Wydawnictwo Medyczne Urban & Partner. Wrocław.

Landau, E., (2001). *Autism*. Franklin Watts, NY

Leonard C., Lombardino L., Mercado L, et al. (1996) Cerebral asymmetry and cognitive development in children: a magnetic resonance imaging study. *Psychological Science* 7: 79-85.

Łojek J., (2006) Pokrojowe uwarunkowania wyboru konia do hipoterapii. *Przegląd Hipoterapeutyczny.*

MacGibbon N.,H., Andrade C.K., Widener. G. Cintas H.L (1998). Effect of an equine-movement therapy program on gait, energy expenditure, and motor function in children with spastic cerebral palsy: a pilot study. *Developmental Medicine and Child Neurology* 40, 754-762

MacKinon, J., Noh, S., Lariveire, J., MacPhail, A., Allan,.D., (1995) Therapeutic horseback riding: A review of the literature. *Physical & Occupational Therapy in Pediatrics*, 15(1), 1-15.

MacKinon, J., Noh, S., Lariveire, J., MacPhail, A., Allan,.D., i Laliberte, D. (1995) A Study of Therapeutic Effects of Horseback Riding for Children with Cerebral Palsy. *Physical & Occupational Therapy in Pediatrics*, 15(1), 17-31.

MacPhail, H.E, Edwards, J.,G., Miller, K., Mosier, C., Zwiers, T., (1998). Trunk Postural Reaction in Children with and Without Cerebral Palsy During Therapeutic Horseback Riding. *Pediatric Physical Theraphy* 10:143-147

Michałowicz. R. red. (1993) *Mózgowe porażenie dziecięce*. Warszawa: Państwowy Zakład Wydawnictw Lekarskich

Miller A, Chretien K. (2007) *The Miller Method. Developing the Capacities of Children on the Autism Spectrum.* Philadelphia: Jessica Kingsley Publishers

Miller A, Eller-Miller E. (1989). *From Ritual to Repertoire. A Cognitive-Developmental Systems Approach with Behavior-Disordered Children.* NY: John Wiley & Sons.

Pisula E., (2002). *Autyzm u dzieci. Diagnoza, klasyfikacje etiologia.* Wydawnictwo Naukowe PWN, Warszawa

Piven & O'Leary, D. (1997). Neuroimaging in autism. *Children and Adolescence Psychiatric Clinics of North America*, 6, 305-323.

Porges, S. (2006). The Vagus: A Mediator of Behavioral and Physiologic Features Associated with Autism. W: Bauman, M., L. I Kemper T., L. red (2006) *The Neurobiology of Autism.* The Johns Hopkins University Press: Baltiomore.

Prizant B., Wetherby A., Rubin E., Laurent A. (2010). *The SCERTS Model.* In ed: Ken Siri, Tony Lyons Cutting Therapies for Autism 2011-2011. Skyhorse Publishing

Przewloka K., (2007) *Synchronization of Sensory Motor Reactions in Children with Autism During Hippotherapy.* Warsaw: University of Physical Education.

Raczek J., Młynarski W., Liach W. (2003) *Kształtowanie i diagnozowanie koordynacyjnych zdolności motorycznych.* AWF Kraków.

Rapi I., Katzman R. (1998) Neurobiology of Autism. *Annals of Neruology* Vol 43: 7-14.

Raun Kaufman (2010). Son-Rise Program In ed: Ken Siri, Tony Lyons *Cutting Therapies for Autism 2011-2011.* Skyhorse Publishing

Rydeen K., (2001) Integration of Sensorimotor and Neurodevelopmental Approches. In: Huebner, R. (2001). *Autism: a sensory motor approach.* (pp.247-261)Maryland: Aspen Publishers' Inc.

Schmahmann, J.D. (1994). The cerebellum in autism: Clinical and anatomical perspectives. In: Bauman, M., L. Kemper T., L. (Eds)).*The Neurobiology of Autism.* (pp. 195-226). Baltimore: The Johns Hopkins University Press.

Shore, S.M., Rastelli, L.G. ((2006). *Understanding Autism for Dummies.* Hoboken, NJ: Wiley Publishing, Inc.

Szopa, J., Mleczko E., Żak S. (1996) *Podstawy Antropomotoryki.* PWN Warszawa –Kraków 1996.

Szot, Z (2004). *Autyzm – terapia ruchowa badania interdyscyplinarne.* AWF Gdańsk.

Waterhouse, L., Fein, D., Modahl, C. (1996) Neurofunctional mechanisms in autism. *Psychological Review,* 103, 457-489.

Winchester P., Kendall, K., Peters, H., Sears, N., Winkley, T., (2002). The Effect of Therapeutic Horseback Riding on Gross Motor Function and Gait Speed in Children Who Are Developmentally Delayed. *Physical & Occupational Therapy in Pediatrics,* 22(3/4), 37-50.

Wingate L., (1982). Feasibility of Horseback Riding as a Therapeutic and Integrative Program for Handicapped Children. *Physical Therapy* 62 (2) 184-186.

Wyżnikiewicz Nawracała, A.(2002) *Jeździectwo w rozwoju motorycznym i psychospołecznym osób niepełnosprawnych.* Gdańsk :AWF Gdańsk

Zabłocki, K.J (2002) *Autyzm.* Wydawnictwo Naukowe Novum, Płock

www.ingramcontent.com/pod-product-compliance
Lightning Source LLC
Chambersburg PA
CBHW072158270326
41930CB00011B/2477